PHLEBOTOMY SOLUTIONS

BACK TO THE BASICS

A GUIDE FOR PHLEBOTOMY STUDENTS

By Al Garza II

Cover by Phlebotomy Solutions 2023

Book Format by Phlebotomy Solutions 2023

ISBN: 978-1-312-14396-8

For questions or comments, please write to

algarza@email.com or

PhlebotomySolutions@email.com

Printed in the United States of America, 2023

Table of Contents

Tales of Phlebotomy

Introduction to Phlebotomy

1. Understanding the Role of a Phlebotomist

Phlebotomy, derived from the Greek words "phlebo" (meaning vein) and "tomy" (meaning to cut), is a crucial healthcare procedure focused on the collection of blood samples for diagnostic testing, transfusions, and research purposes. The role of a phlebotomist is pivotal in the medical field, acting as the bridge between patients and laboratory diagnostics. This section delves into the multifaceted responsibilities and significance of a phlebotomist's role in healthcare.

Key Concepts:

Blood Collection: Phlebotomists are trained professionals responsible for skillfully and safely collecting patient blood specimens. The quality of these specimens directly influences the accuracy of diagnostic tests and subsequent medical decisions.

Patient Interaction: Phlebotomists often interact directly with patients during blood collection. Establishing rapport, demonstrating empathy, and alleviating patient anxiety contribute to a positive patient experience.

Healthcare Team Collaboration: Phlebotomists collaborate closely with nurses, doctors, and laboratory technicians to ensure seamless patient care. Accurate communication and timely specimen delivery are vital to this collaborative effort.

Infection Control: Maintaining strict infection control practices is paramount to prevent the transmission of infections between patients, phlebotomists, and healthcare staff. Adhering to proper protocols safeguards everyone involved.

Ethical Considerations: The collection of blood specimens requires adherence to ethical principles such as patient confidentiality, informed consent, and respecting patient autonomy. Phlebotomists must navigate these considerations with professionalism and sensitivity.

Career Outlook:

The demand for skilled phlebotomists continues to rise as healthcare systems expand and diagnostic capabilities advance. Phlebotomists find employment opportunities in hospitals, clinics, laboratories, blood donation centers, and research institutions. This chapter provides a glimpse into the promising career prospects that await those pursuing a career in phlebotomy.

Conclusion:

Understanding the multifaceted role of a phlebotomist is essential for students aspiring to excel in the field. As guardians of accurate specimen collection, phlebotomists contribute significantly to the healthcare process, enabling accurate diagnoses and informed medical decisions. By mastering the techniques, communication skills, and ethical principles associated with phlebotomy, individuals can embark on a rewarding career dedicated to improving patient care and outcomes.

2. Importance of Phlebotomy in Healthcare

Phlebotomy, the art and science of blood collection, is pivotal in modern healthcare by providing essential diagnostic information and contributing to patient care in diverse medical settings. This section explores the profound importance of phlebotomy and its impact on healthcare practices and outcomes.

Diagnostic Insights:

Phlebotomy serves as the primary means of obtaining blood specimens for diagnostic testing. These specimens enable healthcare professionals to assess a patient's health, diagnose illnesses, monitor disease progression, and tailor treatment plans. Blood tests reveal valuable information about blood cell counts, chemical compositions, and markers of various medical conditions, aiding in early disease detection and effective management.

Evidence-Based Medicine:

The information derived from blood samples collected through phlebotomy drives evidence-based medicine. Physicians and healthcare providers rely on accurate laboratory results to make informed decisions about patient treatment strategies, medication adjustments, and surgical interventions. This reliance on objective data enhances the precision and effectiveness of medical care.

Chronic Disease Management:

Patients with chronic conditions such as diabetes, heart disease, and kidney disorders require frequent monitoring of their health status. Phlebotomy facilitates routine testing, enabling healthcare professionals to monitor changes in disease markers, assess treatment efficacy, and adjust patients' management plans.

Patient Safety and Care:

Accurate and timely blood collection contributes to patient safety by reducing the risk of misdiagnosis and improper treatment. Phlebotomists ensure that collected specimens are correctly labeled, handled, and transported to maintain integrity and prevent errors that could compromise patient care.

Research and Medical Advancements:

Blood samples collected through phlebotomy are invaluable resources for medical research. They contribute to developing new diagnostic tools, medications, and treatment modalities. Research studies based on blood samples help uncover the underlying mechanisms of diseases, leading to breakthroughs in understanding and treating various health conditions.

Emergency Medicine and Critical Care:

In emergencies, phlebotomy assists in rapid diagnosis and treatment decisions. Blood samples obtained from critically ill patients provide real-time information about their condition, aiding medical teams in delivering timely interventions and improving patient outcomes.

Blood Donation and Transfusion:

Phlebotomists play a crucial role in blood donation centers, ensuring the safe collection of blood from donors. Blood transfusions, essential for patients undergoing surgery, experiencing trauma, or dealing with blood disorders, depend on accurately matched blood types, which phlebotomists help identify and crossmatch.

Conclusion:

The importance of phlebotomy in healthcare is far-reaching, impacting diagnosis, treatment, research, and patient safety. As a bridge between patients and medical information, phlebotomy contributes to individual patient care and advances medical science. Understanding the integral role of phlebotomy underscores its significance in ensuring accurate diagnoses, effective treatments, and improved overall health outcomes for patients worldwide.

3. Ethical and Legal Considerations in Phlebotomy

Phlebotomists play a vital role in the healthcare system, collecting blood specimens and contributing to accurate diagnoses and treatment plans. This section delves into the ethical and legal considerations that guide the practice of phlebotomy, ensuring patient rights, safety, and confidentiality are upheld.

Patient Consent and Autonomy:

Respecting patients' autonomy is a cornerstone of ethical phlebotomy practice. Before collecting blood, phlebotomists must obtain informed consent from patients, explaining the procedure, purpose of the blood draw, potential risks, and benefits. Patients can decline or consent to the procedure based on understanding the information provided.

Confidentiality and Privacy:

Maintaining patient confidentiality is of utmost importance. Phlebotomists must ensure that patient information, including test results, medical history, and personal identifiers, remains confidential and is only shared with authorized individuals involved in patient care. This commitment safeguards patients' privacy and builds trust within the healthcare system.

Professionalism and Communication:

Ethical phlebotomists demonstrate professionalism when interacting with patients, colleagues, and other healthcare professionals. Effective communication, empathy, and a respectful demeanor contribute to a positive patient experience and foster trust in the healthcare provider-patient relationship.

Infection Control and Safety:

Adhering to strict infection control practices is both an ethical and legal obligation. Phlebotomists must protect patients and themselves from the transmission of infections by following proper hand hygiene, wearing appropriate personal protective equipment (PPE), and using sterile techniques during blood collection.

Error Prevention and Accuracy:

Ethical phlebotomists prioritize accuracy in specimen collection and labeling to prevent errors that could compromise patient care. Diligent attention to detail reduces the risk of misdiagnosis, inappropriate treatment, and adverse patient outcomes.

Legal Regulations and Scope of Practice:

Phlebotomists must operate within the legal framework defined by their state or country. Understanding their scope of practice, including the specific tasks they are authorized to perform, helps phlebotomists avoid legal pitfalls and ensures they practice safely and effectively.

Informed Refusal and Vulnerable Populations:

Some patients may refuse blood collection due to religious beliefs, personal reasons, or fear. Ethical phlebotomists respect these decisions while providing patients with comprehensive information about the implications of their choices. Additionally, phlebotomists working with vulnerable populations, such as pediatric or elderly patients, should prioritize their comfort and emotional well-being.

Documentation and Record-Keeping:
Accurate and detailed documentation of each blood collection procedure is essential for ethical and legal reasons. Properly labeled specimens, documented consent forms, and clear records contribute to continuity of care, quality assurance, and accountability.

Conclusion:
Ethical and legal considerations are integral to phlebotomy, shaping how phlebotomists interact with patients, collect specimens, and contribute to healthcare. Upholding ethical principles and complying with legal regulations ensures patient rights and safety and elevates the reputation of the phlebotomy profession as a cornerstone of quality healthcare delivery.

4. Anatomy and Physiology for Phlebotomists

Phlebotomists have a fundamental understanding of human anatomy and physiology, essential for safe and adequate blood collection procedures. This section delves into the critical aspects of anatomy and physiology that phlebotomists need to grasp to excel in their field.

Cardiovascular System Overview:
Understanding the cardiovascular system is paramount for phlebotomists, as it involves the network of veins, arteries, and the

heart that transport blood throughout the body. This section explores the anatomy of the heart, its chambers, valves, and the circulatory pathways that carry oxygenated and deoxygenated blood.

Blood Composition and Functions:
Phlebotomists must comprehend the composition of blood, which consists of plasma, red blood cells, white blood cells, and platelets. Learning about the functions of these components, such as oxygen transport, immune response, and clotting, provides context for the importance of blood collection for diagnostic and therapeutic purposes.

Veins and Arteries Relevant to Phlebotomy:
A thorough grasp of veins and arteries is crucial for successful blood collection. Phlebotomists learn to identify and differentiate between veins and arteries, focusing on veins suitable for venipuncture and exploring key locations such as antecubital, cephalic, and basilic veins, which aids in effective blood collection.

Blood Flow and Circulation:
Phlebotomists delve into the concepts of blood flow, circulation, and hemodynamics. Understanding factors influencing blood pressure, velocity, and vessel dilation helps phlebotomists make informed decisions during blood collection procedures.

Vascular Access Devices and Techniques:

In this section, phlebotomists learn about various vascular access devices for blood collection, such as needles, butterfly needles, and intravenous catheters. Mastery of these devices and techniques ensures efficient and minimally discomforting blood draws.

Anatomical Considerations in Venipuncture:

Anatomical variations play a significant role in phlebotomy. Phlebotomists explore factors like vein size, depth, visibility, and considerations for special populations, such as pediatric and geriatric patients.

Hematopoietic System:

Understanding the hematopoietic system, responsible for blood cell production, aids phlebotomists in comprehending the origins and functions of various blood components. Knowledge of bone marrow, erythropoiesis, and leukopoiesis enhances their ability to interpret blood test results accurately.

Conclusion:

A solid foundation in anatomy and physiology is essential for phlebotomists to perform blood collection procedures with precision and care. Phlebotomists ensure patient safety, accurate specimen collection, and a deeper understanding of their role by comprehending the cardiovascular system, blood composition, vascular access techniques, and anatomical considerations.

Overview of the Cardiovascular System

Overview of the Cardiovascular System:

The cardiovascular or circulatory system is a complex network of organs, vessels, and components that transport blood. Comprising the heart, blood vessels, and blood itself, this system plays a crucial role in maintaining oxygen and nutrient supply, waste removal, immune response, and homeostasis.

Heart Anatomy and Function:

The heart, a muscular organ, is divided into four chambers: the right and left atria (upper chambers) and the right and left ventricles (lower chambers). Through a series of coordinated contractions, the heart pumps oxygenated blood to the body's tissues and deoxygenated blood to the lungs for oxygenation.

Blood Vessels:

Blood vessels form pathways through which blood flows. Arteries carry oxygenated blood from the heart to the body's tissues, while veins transport deoxygenated blood back to the heart. Capillaries, tiny vessels, facilitate the exchange of gases, nutrients, and waste products between the blood and surrounding tissues.

1. Blood Composition and Function:

Blood is a complex fluid with different elements that perform essential bodily functions.

1. Plasma: Plasma is the liquid component of blood, accounting for about 55% of its volume. It contains water, electrolytes, proteins, hormones, and waste products. Plasma plays a role in maintaining blood pressure, transporting nutrients, and eliminating waste.

2. Red Blood Cells (Erythrocytes): Red blood cells transport oxygen. They contain hemoglobin, a protein that binds to oxygen in the lungs and releases it to tissues throughout the body. Erythrocytes give blood its characteristic red color.

3. White Blood Cells (Leukocytes): White blood cells are crucial immune system components. They defend the body against infections, bacteria, viruses, and other foreign invaders. Different types of white blood cells have specific functions, including phagocytosis and antibody production.

4. Platelets (Thrombocytes): Platelets are small cell fragments that play a key role in blood clotting (hemostasis). When a blood vessel is injured, platelets aggregate at the site and release substances that initiate clot formation to prevent excessive bleeding.

Blood Functions:
The functions of blood are diverse and vital for maintaining overall health:

1. Oxygen and Nutrient Transport: Red blood cells carry oxygen from the lungs to body tissues and transport nutrients from digestion to cells for energy production.

2. Waste Removal: Blood carries waste products such as carbon dioxide to the lungs for exhalation and transports other waste materials to organs for elimination.

3. Immune Response: White blood cells identify and neutralize pathogens, contributing to the body's defense against infections and diseases.

4. Hormone Transport: Blood transports hormones produced by endocrine glands to target tissues, regulating various bodily functions.

Temperature Regulation: Blood helps regulate body temperature by distributing heat generated by metabolic processes.

pH Balance and Homeostasis: Blood maintains the body's pH within a narrow range, ensuring optimal conditions for enzymatic reactions and overall physiological balance.

Conclusion:

Understanding the composition and functions of blood is essential for phlebotomists, as they collect blood specimens that provide invaluable diagnostic information. Mastery of these concepts enables phlebotomists to comprehend the significance of blood tests, interpret results accurately, and contribute effectively to patient care within the broader context of the cardiovascular system.

2. Veins and Arteries Relevant to Phlebotomy

Phlebotomists require a comprehensive understanding of veins and arteries to execute successful and safe blood collection procedures. This chapter delves into the veins and arteries relevant to phlebotomy, emphasizing their identification, characteristics, and importance in the blood collection.

Vein Identification:

Effective venipuncture relies on identifying suitable veins for blood collection. The antecubital fossa, located in the bend of the arm, is a common site due to its accessibility and prominence. Essential veins in this area include the following:

1. Median Cubital Vein: The median cubital vein connects the cephalic and basilic veins, often appearing as a bridge. It is well-suited for venipuncture due to its consistent location and reduced risk of nerve damage. This is the first vein to locate.

2. Cephalic Vein: Located laterally, the cephalic vein is often the second choice for blood collection due to its visibility and ease of access.

3. Basilic Vein: Positioned medially, the basilic vein is the last
    option. It may be selected when the median or cephalic vein
    is unsuitable or not visible.

Vein Characteristics:

Phlebotomists should consider vein characteristics before
venipuncture:

- Vein Size: Larger veins are typically easier to access and less
  likely to collapse during blood collection.
- Vein Depth: Vein depth varies among individuals.
  Superficial veins are more accessible, while deep veins may
  require advanced techniques.
- Vein Resilience: Some veins are more resilient than others.
  Assessing vein resilience helps prevent complications during
  venipuncture.
- Arterial Avoidance: Phlebotomists must distinguish veins
  from arteries to prevent accidental arterial puncture. Arterial
  blood is oxygenated and pulsates, while venous blood is
  deoxygenated and flows consistently. Pulsation, location, and
  thickness aid in differentiation.

Additional Considerations: Special populations and alternative
sites require specific knowledge:

A. Pediatric Patients: Veins in pediatric patients are smaller and
    more delicate. The dorsal hand veins and feet may be
    considered for blood collection.

B. Geriatric Patients: Aging may cause vein fragility and decreased visibility. Forearm veins are often preferred in geriatric patients.

C. Difficult Veins: Some patients have challenging veins due to obesity, dehydration, or medical conditions. Utilizing warming techniques, proper tourniquet application, and alternative sites can aid in these situations.

Conclusion:

Mastery of veins and arteries relevant to phlebotomy is pivotal for successful blood collection. Phlebotomists ensure patient comfort, specimen quality, and procedural safety by accurately identifying suitable veins, understanding their characteristics, and recognizing arterial differentiation. Adaptability to special populations and considering alternative sites further enhance the phlebotomist's ability to provide optimal patient care.

3. Infection Control and Safety

In phlebotomy, maintaining strict infection control practices and prioritizing safety is paramount to ensure the well-being of patients and healthcare workers. This chapter explores the essential principles and measures of infection control and safety that phlebotomists must adhere to throughout their practice.

Principles of Infection Prevention:

Effective infection control involves following established principles to minimize the risk of spreading infections:

Hand Hygiene: Thorough Handwashing with soap and water or using alcohol-based hand sanitizers before and after each patient interaction is a cornerstone of infection prevention.

Personal Protective Equipment (PPE): Wearing appropriate PPE, such as gloves, gowns, masks, and protective eyewear, provides a barrier against potentially infectious materials.

Respiratory Hygiene/Cough Etiquette: Properly covering the mouth and nose during coughing or sneezing and promptly disposing of tissues help prevent the spread of respiratory infections.

Environmental Cleaning: Regular cleaning and disinfection of equipment, surfaces, and work areas contribute to a clean and safe environment.

Personal Protective Equipment (PPE) Usage:

Phlebotomists must utilize PPE effectively to safeguard themselves and their patients:

1. Gloves: Wearing disposable gloves prevents contact with blood and other potentially infectious materials. Gloves

should be changed between patients and whenever contamination is suspected.

2. Gowns: Protective gowns shield clothing from contamination during procedures involving splashes or sprays of blood or bodily fluids.

3. Masks and Eyewear: Protective eyewear prevents respiratory droplets and splashes from reaching the mouth, nose, and eyes.

4. Proper Handwashing Techniques:

5. Thorough Handwashing is crucial to prevent the transmission of infections:

   a) Wet hands with clean, running water.

   b) Apply soap and rub hands together to create a lather.

   c) Scrub all surfaces of hands, including between fingers and under nails, for at least 20 seconds.

   d) Rinse hands thoroughly under running water.

   e) Dry hands using a clean towel or air dryer.

   f) Standard Precautions and Transmission-Based Precautions:

   g) Standard precautions involve treating all blood and body fluids as potentially infectious. Transmission-based precautions, such as contact, droplet, and airborne precautions, are used when dealing with specific infections.

Needlestick and Sharps Safety:

Proper disposal of needles and other sharps reduces the risk of accidental needlestick injuries. Using safety-engineered devices and designated sharps containers minimizes exposure to contaminated sharps.

Infection Outbreak Control:

In infection outbreaks, phlebotomists play a role in adhering to protocols for preventing the spread of infectious diseases within healthcare settings.

Conclusion:

Infection control and safety are non-negotiable aspects of phlebotomy practice. By following stringent guidelines, utilizing personal protective equipment, practicing proper hand hygiene, and taking precautions to prevent needlestick injuries, phlebotomists contribute to a safe healthcare environment for patients and healthcare providers. These measures protect against infections and uphold the ethical responsibility of providing quality patient care.

Principles of Infection Prevention

In healthcare, the diligent prevention of infections is an essential pillar that underpins patient safety, quality care, and the overall well-being of healthcare providers and those seeking medical attention. The Principles of Infection Prevention are a set of fundamental guidelines that dictate best practices and strategies to minimize the transmission of infections within healthcare settings. These principles are a critical foundation for maintaining a safe environment, upholding ethical standards, and ensuring optimal patient outcomes.

Infection prevention extends beyond the boundaries of any single medical specialty, touching every facet of healthcare practice, from the most intricate surgical procedures to routine patient interactions. The goal is clear: to break the chain of infection transmission and protect vulnerable populations from preventable harm. This involves a comprehensive understanding of infectious agents, modes of transmission, personal protective measures, and environmental control.

Throughout this section, we will delve into the core tenets of infection prevention, exploring the significance of hand hygiene, the proper use of personal protective equipment (PPE), the importance of respiratory hygiene, and the role of environmental cleaning in maintaining a sanitized workspace. By mastering these principles, healthcare providers, including phlebotomists, contribute to the collective effort to create a safer healthcare environment, instill trust in patient-provider relationships, and uphold the ethical commitment to delivering high-quality care.

Understanding and applying the Principles of Infection Prevention not only safeguards patients and providers from the risks associated with infections but also establishes a strong foundation upon which the entire healthcare system relies. Through their commitment to these principles, healthcare professionals demonstrate their dedication to excellence, compassion, and the pursuit of a healthier future for all.

1. Personal Protective Equipment (PPE) Usage

Personal Protective Equipment (PPE) is a crucial barrier between healthcare providers and potentially infectious materials, safeguarding the provider and the patient. In the context of phlebotomy and various healthcare procedures, understanding the appropriate selection, proper usage, and correct disposal of PPE is essential to prevent the transmission of infections. This section delves into the critical aspects of PPE usage, highlighting its significance and practical implementation.

Selecting the Right PPE: Choosing the appropriate PPE depends on the nature of the task and the potential for exposure to infectious agents. Common types of PPE include:

- **Gloves:** Disposable gloves create a barrier between hands and potential contaminants. They are essential for all patient interactions, mainly when contacting blood or bodily fluids.
- **Gowns:** Protective gowns shield clothing from splashes, sprays, and contamination during procedures that carry a risk of exposure.
- **Masks and Protective Eyewear:** Masks prevent inhaling respiratory droplets only, while protective eyewear shields the eyes from splashes and airborne particles.

Proper PPE Usage: Adhering to proper PPE usage guidelines is vital for infection prevention:

- **Gloves:** Wear gloves when touching blood, body fluids, mucous membranes, or non-intact skin. Change gloves between patients, after contamination, and when moving from a contaminated to a clean area.
- **Gowns:** Put on a gown when there is a potential for a splash or spray of blood, bodily fluids, or other contaminants. Remove the gown carefully and dispose of it appropriately after use.
- **Masks and Eyewear:** Wear masks and protective eyewear when performing procedures that might generate respiratory droplets or expose the eyes to splashes.

Donning and Doffing PPE: Correctly donning (putting on) and doffing (taking off) PPE is critical to prevent contamination:

Donning:
1. Wash hands thoroughly before donning PPE.
2. Put on a gown (if needed) and secure it at the back.
3. Don gloves, ensuring they cover wrists and gown cuffs.

Doffing:
1. Remove gloves by peeling them off inside-out, starting from the wrist.
2. Untie and remove the gown, rolling it inside out as you do so.
3. Perform hand hygiene.
4. Remove eyewear and mask by touching only the designated areas (ear loops or ties).
5. Rewash hands after doffing PPE.

PPE Disposal: Proper disposal of PPE is crucial to prevent the spread of contamination:

- **Gloves and Gowns:** Discard gloves and gowns into designated waste containers immediately after use.
- **Masks and Eyewear:** Place used masks and eyewear in appropriate waste containers. Do not touch the front of the mask during removal.

Conclusion: Personal Protective Equipment is an integral aspect of infection control in phlebotomy and healthcare. Proper PPE usage ensures the safety of both healthcare providers and patients, minimizing the risk of infection transmission. By understanding the correct selection, donning, doffing, and disposal of PPE, phlebotomists contribute to a safe healthcare environment and uphold the highest standards of patient care.

2. Proper Handwashing Techniques

Hand hygiene is fundamental to infection prevention and control in healthcare settings. Effective handwashing techniques are essential for healthcare providers, including phlebotomists, to reduce the risk of transmitting infections to patients and colleagues. This section outlines the importance of proper handwashing techniques and provides step-by-step guidance for thorough hand hygiene.

Why Handwashing Matters: Hands are a standard route for transmitting microorganisms, including bacteria, viruses, and other pathogens. Proper Handwashing breaks the chain of infection transmission and plays a pivotal role in safeguarding patients and healthcare providers from potential harm.

When to Wash Hands: Phlebotomists should perform hand hygiene in various situations, including:

- Before and after patient contact
- Before and after putting on or removing gloves

- After touching contaminated surfaces or objects

- After using the restroom

- Before eating or handling food

Steps for Effective Handwashing:

1. **Wet Hands:** Use clean, running water to wet your hands thoroughly.

2. **Apply Soap:** Apply an adequate amount of soap to your hands.

3. **Lather:** Rub your hands together to create a lather. Ensure that you cover all surfaces, including the backs of your hands, between your fingers, and under your nails.

4. **Scrub for 20 Seconds:** Scrub your hands for at least 20 seconds. You can use a timer or hum the "Happy Birthday" song twice to gauge the appropriate duration.

5. **Rinse Thoroughly:** Rinse your hands under clean, running water, removing all soap.

6. **Dry Hands:** Dry your hands using a clean towel or air dryer. Use a disposable towel to turn off the faucet and open the door if possible.

Special Considerations:

- **Hand Jewelry:** Remove hand jewelry before Handwashing, as pathogens can accumulate under rings and other jewelry.

- **Nail Care:** Keep nails short and clean to prevent harboring microorganisms.

- **Hand Creams:** Use hand creams to prevent dryness and cracking, but avoid using them immediately before providing patient care.

Alcohol-Based Hand Sanitizers: When soap and water are not readily available, alcohol-based hand sanitizers can be used:

1. Apply an appropriate amount of sanitizer to the palm of one hand.
2. Rub your hands together, covering all surfaces, until they feel dry.

Conclusion: Proper handwashing techniques are a simple yet powerful means of infection prevention for phlebotomists and all healthcare providers. By making thorough hand hygiene a routine practice, phlebotomists contribute to a safe healthcare environment, protect patients from infections, and uphold the highest standards of patient care.

3. Equipment and Supplies

In phlebotomy, a comprehensive understanding of the equipment and supplies used in blood collection procedures is essential for ensuring patient safety, specimen integrity, and the overall success of the process. This section delves into the critical components of equipment and supplies utilized by phlebotomists, providing insights into their functions, proper usage, and importance in the field.

Phlebotomy procedures use specialized equipment to facilitate safe and efficient blood collection. Understanding the purpose and proper utilization of each piece of equipment is vital for maintaining the quality of specimens.

Types of Collection Tubes and Additives: Collection tubes come in various sizes and colors, each serving a specific purpose in blood collection and testing. These tubes may contain additives that preserve the integrity of the collected blood and aid in performing specific laboratory tests.

Needle Gauges and Selection: Needles used in phlebotomy procedures vary in size, with different gauges suited for different situations. Needle gauge selection depends on the patient's vein size, the blood draw's purpose, and the blood's viscosity.

Venipuncture Devices: Needles vs. Butterflies: Phlebotomists can choose between standard needles and butterfly needles (winged infusion sets) for venipuncture. Butterfly needles are particularly useful when working with small or fragile veins, offering better control and reduced discomfort.

Blood Culture Collection and Techniques: Blood culture collection is crucial for diagnosing bloodstream infections. Proper technique, sterile equipment, and blood culture bottles with specific additives provide accurate results and guide appropriate treatment.

Considerations for Safe Equipment Usage: Maintaining patient safety and specimen integrity involves adhering to several considerations:

- Proper equipment disinfection or sterilization before use.
- Correct labeling of collection tubes to prevent errors.
- Applying tourniquets and selecting appropriate veins for venipuncture.
- Ensuring needles are inserted at the proper angle and depth.

Safety Devices and Needlestick Prevention: Needlestick injuries are a significant risk for healthcare providers. Safety-engineered devices, including needles with retractable mechanisms, help reduce the likelihood of accidental needlestick injuries during and after venipuncture.

Conclusion: A thorough understanding of phlebotomy equipment and supplies is indispensable for the safe and effective execution of blood collection procedures. By mastering the nuances of collection tubes, additives, needle selection, and safe device usage, phlebotomists ensure the accuracy of laboratory tests, minimize patient discomfort, and uphold the highest standards of patient care.

Introduction to Phlebotomy Equipment

Phlebotomy, the art of blood collection, is a precise and intricate procedure that requires a specialized set of equipment designed to ensure patient safety, specimen quality, and the accuracy of diagnostic testing. The section "Introduction to Phlebotomy Equipment" offers a comprehensive overview of the essential tools utilized by phlebotomists in their daily practice. This section dives into the foundational components that enable phlebotomists to perform their roles with precision and care, from collection tubes to needles and venipuncture devices.

Each piece of phlebotomy equipment serves a specific purpose, whether collecting blood samples for diagnostic purposes, maintaining sample integrity during transportation, or minimizing the risk of complications for the healthcare provider and the patient. Understanding the functions, proper usage, and benefits of different types of equipment is paramount for any phlebotomist aiming to excel in their profession.

By immersing themselves in the world of phlebotomy equipment, phlebotomists gain a deeper appreciation for the intricacies of their field and the impact their work has on patient care. From the moment a blood sample is drawn to its journey through the laboratory, the equipment used plays a pivotal role in delivering accurate diagnoses and improving healthcare outcomes.

As we delve into the nuances of phlebotomy equipment, let us explore the significance of each tool, its role in the blood collection process, and the best practices for its usage. With this knowledge, phlebotomists can confidently navigate the equipment world, ensuring that each blood collection procedure is conducted with the highest professionalism, precision, and patient-centered care.

1. Types of Collection Tubes and Additives

The process of blood collection in phlebotomy is not merely about drawing blood but also about preserving the sample's integrity for accurate diagnostic testing. One of the critical aspects of achieving this goal involves using different collection tubes, each designed to serve a specific purpose in the blood collection process. This section delves into the various types of collection tubes and the additives they contain, shedding light on their significance and contributions to successful phlebotomy practices.

Introduction to Collection Tubes and Additives: Collection tubes are essential tools in phlebotomy, as they play a pivotal role in maintaining the quality of blood samples and facilitating the performance of various laboratory tests. These tubes are designed with specific additives that prevent blood coagulation, stabilize analytes, and enhance the accuracy of diagnostic results.

Types of Collection Tubes: Different types of collection tubes are color-coded to indicate the specific tests they are suitable for:

1. **Red Top Tubes:** These tubes lack additives and allow blood to clot naturally. Serum collected from these tubes is used for chemistry tests, serology, and blood bank testing.

2. **Light Blue Top Tubes:** These tubes contain sodium citrate, which prevents blood clotting by binding to calcium. They are primarily used for coagulation studies and clotting factor tests.

3. **Green Top Tubes:** Containing heparin, these tubes are used for plasma tests that require anticoagulated blood samples, such as electrolyte analyses and blood gas testing.

4. **Lavender Top Tubes:** Containing the anticoagulant EDTA, these tubes are used for hematology tests and blood cell count analyses.

5. **Gray Top Tubes:** These tubes contain sodium fluoride, which preserves glucose levels and inhibits glycolysis. They are commonly used for glucose and lactate testing.

***NOTE**: Blood Cultures are always first in the order of draw. SST and PST tubes are used after Light Blue in the order of draw. SST=Serum Separater and PST=Plasma Separater Tubes.

The Role of Additives: The additives present in collection tubes serve specific purposes:

*   **Anticoagulants:** Prevent blood clotting by inhibiting coagulation factors or binding calcium ions.

- **Preservatives:** Stabilize specific analytes to prevent changes in sample composition over time.
- **Gel Separators:** These substances help separate serum or plasma from blood cells, facilitating the separation process during centrifugation.

Selecting the Right Tube: Phlebotomists must accurately select the appropriate collection tube based on the required tests. Incorrect tube selection can lead to inaccurate results, compromised patient care, and even death.

Conclusion: Understanding the collection tube types and their respective additives is fundamental to phlebotomy. By selecting the proper tube for each blood collection procedure, phlebotomists contribute to the accuracy of diagnostic testing, ensuring that patients receive reliable results that guide effective medical decisions. Mastery of collection tubes and additives is a testament to the commitment of phlebotomists to delivering the highest standards of patient care.

2. Needle Gauges and Selection

Needles are integral tools in phlebotomy, serving as the conduit through which blood is collected from patients. The gauge of a needle, denoting its diameter, plays a crucial role in determining the patient's comfort and the efficiency of blood collection. This section delves into the concept of needle gauges, their importance, and the factors influencing the selection of the appropriate needle gauge for blood collection procedures.

Understanding Needle Gauges: A needle gauge is a diameter typically measured in numbers. Smaller gauge numbers represent larger needle diameters, while larger gauge numbers indicate thinner needles. Needle gauges commonly used in phlebotomy range from 21 to 23, with 21 being the thickest and 23 the thinnest.

Importance of Needle Gauge Selection: Selecting the appropriate needle gauge is essential for several reasons:

- **Patient Comfort:** Thicker needles (lower gauge numbers) are less likely to cause pain during insertion, making them suitable for patients with more prominent veins.
- **Vein Size:** The size of the patient's veins influences needle gauge selection. Larger veins can accommodate thicker needles, while smaller veins require thinner needles.
- **Viscosity of Blood:** Blood viscosity affects the ease of blood flow through the needle. Thicker needles are more effective for drawing viscous blood.
- **Blood Collection Purpose:** Blood collection also influences needle gauge selection. For routine blood tests, a standard needle gauge may suffice. However, specialized tests or blood cultures might require specific gauges.

Commonly Used Needle Gauges:

- **21-Gauge Needle:** This standard needle gauge is often used for routine blood collection. It strikes a balance between patient comfort and adequate blood flow.
- **23-Gauge Needle:** Thinner needles like the 23-gauge are commonly used for procedures requiring minimal blood collection or for patients with delicate veins.
- **25-Gauge Needle:** The 25-gauge needle was among the thinnest and was used for special situations, such as drawing blood from pediatric patients. However, this needle has now been discontinued due to hemolysis of the blood. The needle is too small for proper blood collection.

Factors Influencing Needle Gauge Selection: Several factors guide the selection of the appropriate needle gauge:

- **Patient Age:** Pediatric and geriatric patients often require thinner needles due to smaller veins and skin fragility.
- **Procedure Type:** The purpose of the blood collection, whether for routine tests, blood cultures, or specialized assays, affects needle gauge choice.
- **Vein Accessibility:** The size and visibility of the patient's veins impact the needle gauge that can be safely used.

Conclusion: Selecting the correct needle gauge is a nuanced decision that requires consideration of patient comfort, vein size, blood viscosity, and the specific blood collection purpose. By understanding these factors and making informed needle gauge selections, phlebotomists contribute to patient satisfaction, efficient blood collection, and the overall success of the phlebotomy procedure.

3. Venipuncture Devices: Needles vs. Butterfly

Venipuncture, the process of puncturing a vein to collect blood, is a core skill in phlebotomy. Phlebotomists have the option to choose between different venipuncture devices, including standard needles and butterfly needles (winged infusion sets). This section explores the characteristics, benefits, and considerations associated with each type of venipuncture device, enabling phlebotomists to make informed decisions based on patient needs and procedural requirements.

Standard Needles:

Standard needles, also known as straight needles, are the traditional choice for venipuncture. These needles are commonly used due to their simplicity and versatility.

Benefits of Standard Needles:

- **Direct Insertion:** Standard needles offer direct insertion into the vein, making them suitable for patients with visible and easily accessible veins.
- **Familiarity:** Phlebotomists are often trained to use standard needles from the outset of their careers.
- **Various Sizes:** Standard needles are available in various sizes, allowing phlebotomists to choose the most appropriate gauge for each patient.

Considerations for Standard Needles:

- **Patient Comfort:** Some patients may experience discomfort during insertion, especially if the veins are delicate or difficult to access.
- **Limited Control:** While standard needles provide control during insertion, they may be challenging to control once inside the vein due to their length.

Butterfly Needles (Winged Infusion Sets):

Butterfly needles, also known as winged infusion sets or "butterfly sets," are specialized venipuncture devices that offer distinct advantages in specific situations.

Benefits of Butterfly Needles:

- **Delicate Veins:** Butterfly needles are particularly useful for patients with small, fragile, or difficult-to-access veins.

- **Controlled Insertion:** The smaller size and design of butterfly needles provide better control during insertion, reducing the risk of complications.

- **Less Discomfort:** Due to their smaller gauge and gentler insertion, butterfly needles often cause less discomfort to patients.

- **Pediatric and Geriatric Patients:** Butterfly needles are preferred for pediatric and geriatric patients due to their reduced risk of vein damage.

Considerations for Butterfly Needles:

- **Blood Flow:** Butterfly needles may have a slightly slower blood flow rate than standard needles, making them better suited for smaller blood volume collections.

- **Length of Use:** Butterfly needles are ideal for short-term collections, as their small size may hinder their suitability for prolonged procedures.

Choosing the Appropriate Device: Phlebotomists must consider patient factors, vein accessibility, and procedural requirements when selecting between standard needles and butterfly needles. Utilizing both devices in their practice allows phlebotomists to tailor their approach to ensuring patient comfort and specimen quality.

Conclusion: The choice between standard needles and butterfly needles in venipuncture depends on factors such as patient comfort, vein accessibility, and the purpose of the blood collection. By understanding the benefits and considerations of each venipuncture device, phlebotomists enhance their ability to provide efficient, patient-centered care and ensure the success of blood collection procedures.

4. Blood Culture Collection and Techniques

Blood culture collection is a specialized aspect of phlebotomy that is important in diagnosing and treating bloodstream infections. Proper technique, sterile equipment, and meticulous attention to detail are essential to ensure accurate and reliable results. This section delves into the intricacies of blood culture collection and techniques, highlighting their role in identifying pathogens responsible for infections and guiding appropriate patient care.

Introduction to Blood Culture Collection: Blood cultures involve the collection of blood samples to identify the presence of microorganisms, such as bacteria or fungi, causing bloodstream infections (bacteremia or fungemia). Timely and accurate blood culture results guide clinicians in selecting the most effective antibiotics for treatment.

Sterility and Aseptic Technique: Maintaining sterility and adhering to aseptic technique during blood culture collection are paramount. Proper hand hygiene, sterile gloves, and sterile equipment prevent blood sample contamination.

Blood Culture Bottle Selection: Blood culture bottles contain specific additives that promote the growth of microorganisms if present in the blood. These bottles are categorized as aerobic (requiring oxygen) or anaerobic (without oxygen) based on the type of microorganisms they support.

Blood Culture Collection Techniques:

1. **Preparation:** Gather the necessary equipment, perform hand hygiene, and assemble sterile supplies.
2. **Select Site:** Identify the appropriate venipuncture site using a sterile technique.
3. **Disinfection:** Clean the venipuncture site with an antiseptic solution, allowing it to dry before proceeding.
4. **Needle Insertion:** Use sterile technique to insert the needle into the vein, ensuring minimal contamination.
5. **Blood Culture Bottle Collection:** Collect the appropriate blood volume into the culture bottles using aseptic technique. Fill the aerobic bottle first, followed by the anaerobic bottle.
6. **Mixing:** Gently invert the culture bottles to mix the blood with the additive.
7. **Labeling:** Label the blood culture bottles with patient

information, date, and time of collection.

8. **Transportation:** Immediately transport the blood culture bottles to the laboratory to initiate incubation and analysis.

Potential Complications and Troubleshooting:

- **Contamination:** Improper technique can introduce contaminants, leading to false-positive results. Strict adherence to sterile practices minimizes this risk.

- **False-Negative Results:** If insufficient blood is collected or the patient has been on antibiotics, the blood culture might yield false-negative results.

Interpreting Blood Culture Results: Laboratory technicians analyze the blood culture bottles for bacterial or fungal growth signs. Positive results indicate the presence of pathogens causing infections, while negative results suggest no active infection at the time of blood collection.

Conclusion: Blood culture collection and techniques are critical for infection diagnosis and treatment. By employing strict aseptic practices, selecting appropriate blood culture bottles, and following precise collection steps, phlebotomists contribute to accurate diagnostic results that guide clinicians in providing targeted and effective patient care. Mastery of blood culture collection techniques underscores the dedication of phlebotomists to patient well-being and upholds the highest standards of infection control.

5. Patient Identification and Communication

Effective patient identification and communication are cornerstones of safe and ethical phlebotomy practice. Accurate patient identification ensures that samples are correctly attributed, while clear communication fosters trust, reduces anxiety, and enhances the overall patient experience. This section delves into the importance of patient identification and communication in phlebotomy, emphasizing best practices for maintaining patient safety and satisfaction.

Patient Identification:

Patient misidentification can lead to severe consequences, including incorrect diagnoses, inappropriate treatments, and compromised patient safety. Ensuring accurate patient identification is a fundamental responsibility of phlebotomists.

Best Practices for Patient Identification:

- **Verify Identity:** Always verify the patient's identity using at least two unique identifiers, such as full name, date of birth, or medical record number.
- **Avoid Assumptions:** Never assume a patient's identity based on appearance. Always ask for confirmation from the patient.
- **Use Technology:** Utilize barcode scanning systems or electronic health records to enhance accuracy in patient identification.

Effective Communication:

Clear and empathetic communication is essential for alleviating patient anxiety, addressing concerns, and establishing a positive rapport. Effective communication also ensures that patients understand the procedures being performed.

Best Practices for Effective Communication:

- **Explain Procedures:** Communicate the purpose of the procedure, the steps involved, and any potential discomfort the patient may experience.
- **Active Listening:** Listen attentively to patients' questions, concerns, and preferences and address them with empathy.
- **Use Layman's Terms:** Avoid medical jargon and use simple, understandable language when explaining patient procedures.
- **Manage Anxiety:** Acknowledge and address patient anxiety by offering reassurance and maintaining a calm demeanor.

Special Considerations:

- **Pediatric Patients:** Use child-friendly language and approach when communicating with pediatric patients. Offer distractions, such as toys or games, to ease anxiety.
- **Elderly Patients:** Speak clearly and allow extra time for elderly patients to process information and ask questions.
- **Language Barriers:** If patients speak a different language, use interpreters or translation services.

Conclusion: Patient identification and communication are integral aspects of phlebotomy practice that contribute to patient safety, trust, and overall satisfaction. By adhering to accurate patient identification protocols and employing effective communication strategies, phlebotomists ensure that patients are treated with the utmost respect, compassion, and professionalism. These practices not only enhance the patient experience but also reflect the commitment of phlebotomists to providing exceptional care in every interaction.

Ensuring Accurate Patient Identification

Accurate patient identification is a critical foundation for safe and effective care delivery in healthcare. Ensuring that each patient is correctly identified is not only a professional responsibility but also a matter of ethical and legal importance. By establishing a robust framework for proper patient identification, phlebotomists contribute to patient safety, trust, and the overall quality of care.

The potential for patient misidentification is ever-present in the fast-paced environment of healthcare facilities, where patients come from diverse backgrounds and conditions. The consequences of such errors can range from diagnostic inaccuracies to unnecessary treatments or delays in providing appropriate care. Therefore, a meticulous approach to confirming patient identity is paramount. Throughout this section, we will explore the essential practices and protocols that phlebotomists should employ to verify the identity of each patient before performing blood collection procedures. Utilizing unique identifiers, leveraging technology, and embracing a culture of vigilance are among the strategies phlebotomists can adopt to prevent misidentification errors.

The commitment to accurate patient identification extends beyond the act of blood collection itself. It is a thread that runs through the entire fabric of healthcare, ensuring that patients receive the right treatments, medications, and interventions. By establishing a solid foundation of accurate patient identification, phlebotomists play a vital role in upholding the principles of patient-centered care, safety, and ethical practice.

1. Effective Communication with Patients

Communication is a cornerstone of effective and compassionate healthcare practice. Regarding phlebotomy, transparent and empathetic communication is pivotal in alleviating patient anxiety, fostering trust, and ensuring a positive patient experience. This section explores the art of effective communication with patients during phlebotomy procedures, highlighting strategies and best practices for building rapport and enhancing patient satisfaction.

Introduction to Effective Communication: Effective communication extends beyond the mere exchange of words—it encompasses active listening, empathy, and a genuine desire to connect with patients on a human level. In phlebotomy, effective communication creates a supportive environment where patients feel respected, informed, and at ease.

Building Rapport: Rapport-building is the foundation of successful patient interactions. Establishing a positive rapport eases patient anxiety and contributes to better cooperation during the procedure.

Strategies for Effective Communication:

1. **Explaining Procedures:** Before beginning the blood collection, explain the procedure in simple language, detailing the steps involved and addressing any patient concerns.

2. **Active Listening:** Pay close attention to the patient's questions, concerns, and preferences. Validate their feelings and show that their thoughts are valued.

3. **Using Empathetic Language:** Express empathy and understanding using phrases like "I understand how you feel" or "I am here to help."

4. **Encouraging Questions:** Encourage patients to ask questions and express their concerns. Answer their queries with patience and clarity.

5. **Maintaining a Calm Demeanor:** Display a calm and reassuring demeanor throughout the procedure. Your demeanor influences the patient's perception of the experience.

6. **Offering Reassurance:** Reassure patients that discomfort will be minimal and temporary. Use positive language to set their expectations.

7. **Acknowledging Anxiety:** Recognize and acknowledge patient anxiety. Assure their feelings are normal and that you are there to support them.

Special Considerations:

- **Pediatric Patients:** Engage pediatric patients with age-appropriate communication, using visual aids and distraction techniques to ease anxiety.

- **Elderly Patients:** Speak clearly and at a moderate pace when communicating with elderly patients. Allow them ample time to process information and ask questions.

- **Language Barriers:** When language barriers exist, use interpreters or translation services to ensure effective communication.

Benefits of Effective Communication: Effective communication during phlebotomy has numerous benefits:

- **Reduced Anxiety:** Clear communication reduces patient anxiety and enhances their overall experience.

- **Trust and Compliance:** Patients are more likely to comply with instructions and follow the procedure when they trust the healthcare provider.

- **Patient-Centered Care:** Effective communication aligns with patient-centered care principles, where patients actively participate in their healthcare journey.

Conclusion: Effective communication is a skill that empowers phlebotomists to establish meaningful connections with patients, provide information, and address concerns. By cultivating strong communication skills, phlebotomists contribute to positive patient experiences, promote patient-centered care, and uphold the core principles of compassionate and ethical healthcare practice.

2. Dealing with Anxious and Difficult Patients

Encountering anxious or difficult patients is a common challenge in healthcare, including phlebotomy. Nervousness, fear, and discomfort can heighten patient anxiety during blood collection procedures, leading to tense interactions. This section addresses strategies for effectively managing anxious and difficult patients, ensuring their comfort, safety, and overall satisfaction while upholding the principles of patient-centered care.

Introduction to Dealing with Anxious and Difficult Patients: Anxiety and difficulty are natural responses in the context of healthcare procedures, and acknowledging and addressing these emotions is vital for delivering high-quality care. As compassionate healthcare professionals, phlebotomists are crucial in creating a supportive environment that eases patient apprehension.

Understanding Patient Anxiety: Anxiety often stems from fear of the unknown, past negative experiences, or discomfort with medical procedures. Recognizing the underlying factors of patient anxiety allows phlebotomists to tailor their approach.

Strategies for Managing Anxious and Difficult Patients:

1. **Empathy and Active Listening:** Show genuine concern and actively listen to patients' concerns. Acknowledge their anxiety and validate their emotions.

2. **Explain Procedures:** Provide a clear, step-by-step explanation of the procedure, addressing any misconceptions or fears they may have.

3. **Offer Choices:** Allow patients to make small choices, such as selecting the arm for blood collection or choosing the order of steps, to give them a sense of control.

4. **Use Distraction Techniques:** Engage patients in conversation about unrelated topics or offer distractions such as visual aids to redirect their focus.

5. **Provide Reassurance:** Reassure patients that the procedure will be quick, relatively painless, and conducted by a skilled professional.

6. **Pause and Address Concerns:** If patients express concerns mid-procedure, pause and address their worries before proceeding.

7. **Nonverbal Communication:** Use a calm and soothing tone of voice, maintain eye contact, and exhibit a relaxed posture to convey empathy and reassurance.

Handling Difficult Patients:

1. **Stay Calm:** Maintain your composure even if a patient becomes difficult or agitated.

2. **Set Boundaries:** Establish clear boundaries and communicate expectations for behavior during the procedure.

3. **Seek Assistance:** If a situation escalates, involve a supervisor or a colleague to provide support.

Special Considerations:

- **Pediatric Patients:** Use child-friendly language, explain using toys or illustrations, and offer comfort items like stuffed animals.

- **Elderly Patients:** Show patience and allow additional time for elderly patients to express their concerns.

- **Phobia Management:** For patients with specific phobias, such as fear of needles (trypanophobia), explore desensitization techniques or consider referral to a specialist.

Benefits of Effective Management: Effectively managing anxious and difficult patients yields numerous benefits:

- **Patient Satisfaction:** Patients appreciate understanding and compassionate care, enhancing their overall satisfaction.

- **Trust Building:** Compassionate and empathetic management builds trust and rapport between patients and healthcare providers.

- **Enhanced Outcomes:** Calming patient anxiety improves cooperation, reduces the likelihood of complications, and ensures accurate sample collection.

Conclusion: Dealing with anxious and difficult patients requires a blend of empathy, communication skills, and patience. By addressing patients' emotional needs, employing effective communication strategies, and tailoring approaches to individual preferences, phlebotomists create a safe and supportive environment that promotes positive patient experiences. Upholding patient-centered care principles, even in challenging situations, reflects the commitment of phlebotomists to the well-being and comfort of their patients.

Steps of Venipuncture Procedure

Venipuncture, the process of puncturing a vein to collect blood, is a fundamental skill in phlebotomy. Proficiency in venipuncture techniques is essential for minimizing patient discomfort, ensuring specimen quality, and maintaining patient safety. This section delves into the intricacies of venipuncture techniques, covering the steps, best practices, and considerations that phlebotomists should master to excel in their practice.

Introduction to Venipuncture Techniques: Venipuncture involves technical proficiency and a comprehensive understanding of patient comfort, vein selection, and proper equipment utilization. Mastery of venipuncture techniques allows phlebotomists to collect blood with precision, confidence, and patient-centered care.

Key Steps in Venipuncture:

1. **Preparation:** Gather necessary equipment, confirm patient identity, and ensure a sterile environment. Ask the patient if they are taking blood-thinners or have gotten dizzy or fainted in the past. Prepare accordingly if they answered yes.

2. **Patient Positioning:** Choose a comfortable and accessible venipuncture site. Position the patient's arm and prepare the tourniquet.

3. **Tourniquet Application:** Apply a tourniquet 3 to 4 inches above the selected venipuncture site to engorge the vein and

make it easier to locate. (1 minute rule.)

4. **Vein Selection:** Palpate the veins to identify the most suitable one for venipuncture. Consider factors such as vein size, depth, and visibility.

5. **Skin Disinfection:** Clean the venipuncture site using an antiseptic solution, allowing it to dry before proceeding.

6. **Needle Insertion:** Insert the needle at a slight angle of 15 to 30 degrees into the selected vein, using a smooth and controlled motion. (hand angle is 5-10 degrees.)

7. **Blood Collection:** Observe the needle for blood flashback in the flashback chamber or tubing, indicating successful needle placement. If no blood flows into the tube, adjust the needle if necessary by going deeper or slowly withdrawing the needle until blood flows. NO FISHING!

8. **Needle Stabilization:** Stabilize the needle with one hand while using the other hand to control the blood collection tubes.

9. **Tube Change:** After filling the initial tube, switch to additional tubes as needed for the requested tests. Remember always to invert each tube to mix the additive with the blood.

10. **Tourniquet Removal:** Remove the tourniquet before bandaging the venipuncture site and before the needle.

11. **Needle Removal:** After blood collection, the needle is withdrawn smoothly, and apply gentle pressure using sterile gauze for 3-5 minutes before checking for hemostasis.

12. **Patient Comfort and Post-Procedure:** Provide patients with post-procedure instructions and ensure their comfort before concluding. Instructions include leaving the bandage on for at least 15 minutes, not bending the elbow, or lifting anything for at least an hour to prevent bruising at the site.

Best Practices and Considerations:

- **Needle Angle:** The needle should be inserted at a shallow angle (15-30 degrees) to the skin's surface to minimize discomfort and improve vein entry.

- **Vein Anchoring:** To prevent vein rolling during insertion, apply gentle pressure above and below the venipuncture site.

- **Releasing Tourniquet:** Release the tourniquet before filling the last tube to prevent blood clotting issues.

- **Appropriate Tube Order:** Collect tubes appropriately to avoid cross-contamination and ensure accurate test results.

Conclusion: Venipuncture techniques are the cornerstone of blood collection procedures in phlebotomy. Phlebotomists ensure successful venipuncture outcomes by mastering the steps, understanding patient comfort, and consistently applying best practices. Proficiency in venipuncture techniques enhances patient experiences, minimizes potential complications, and contributes to the overall delivery of safe and high-quality patient care.

1. Tourniquet Application and Vein Selection

Tourniquet application and vein selection are crucial initial steps in venipuncture, setting the stage for a successful blood collection procedure. These steps influence patient comfort, the visibility of veins, and the ease of needle insertion. This section explores the techniques and considerations for effectively applying a tourniquet and selecting an appropriate vein for venipuncture.

A tourniquet is a constricting band that temporarily restricts blood flow in the veins, making them more prominent and accessible for venipuncture. A tourniquet should never be on a patient for more than 1 minute.

Steps for Tourniquet Application:

1. **Gather Equipment:** Ensure you have an appropriately sized tourniquet and the patient's arm is accessible.

2. **Patient Preparation:** Explain the purpose of the tourniquet to the patient and address any concerns they may have.

3. **Selecting the Site:** Choose a site slightly above the intended venipuncture site, ensuring the tourniquet is not too tight.

4. **Application:** Wrap the tourniquet around the patient's arm and secure it 3-4 inches above the site, leaving enough room to insert a finger underneath. The tourniquet should be snug but not overly tight.

5. **Check for Comfort:** Ensure the patient is comfortable and not experiencing excessive discomfort due to the tourniquet.

6. **Release Timing:** Release the tourniquet after a blood flashback is observed in the needle and blood collection has begun if you have gone over 1 minute.

Considerations for Tourniquet Application:

- **Tourniquet Time:** Avoid leaving the tourniquet on for more than one minute to prevent blood stasis and unnecessary discomfort.
- **Alternate Sites:** If the initial tourniquet application is unsuccessful, release it and try a different location.

Vein Selection:

Choosing an appropriate vein for venipuncture is essential to ensure a successful blood collection procedure and patient comfort.

Considerations for Vein Selection:

1. **Vein Visibility:** Opt for visible and palpable veins, as they are easier to locate and access.
2. **Vein Size:** Select veins of suitable size, considering the gauge of the needle and the volume of blood required.
3. **Vein Accessibility:** Choose veins that are easily accessible and free from obstructions.
4. **Patient Comfort:** Prioritize comfort by avoiding veins over bony areas or nerves.
5. **Dominant Hand:** If possible, choose the non-dominant hand for venipuncture to minimize disruption to daily activities.

Vein Selection Sites:

- **Antecubital Fossa:** Located on the inner arm, this is a common site for venipuncture due to prominent veins. *Always follow the order of veins.*

- **Dorsal Hand Veins:** Suitable for patients with delicate veins or when other sites are not accessible.

- **Wrist Veins:** Used when other sites are challenging, wrist veins should be cautiously approached due to their sensitivity.

- **Foot Veins:** Only used when all other veins listed above are unavailable and only with a doctor's approval or order.

Conclusion: Effective tourniquet application and vein selection set the foundation for a successful venipuncture procedure. By mastering these initial steps, phlebotomists ensure patient comfort, enhance vein visibility and facilitate efficient blood collection. These skills underscore phlebotomists' commitment to patient-centered care, precision, and safe blood collection practices.

2. Complications and Troubleshooting

Even with meticulous technique, complications can arise during the venipuncture process in phlebotomy. Being prepared to identify and address these complications is essential for ensuring patient safety, obtaining accurate samples, and maintaining the integrity of the blood collection procedure. This section explores potential complications, their causes, and troubleshooting strategies that phlebotomists should be well-versed in to handle unforeseen challenges effectively. Understanding that complications can occur is fundamental to safe and responsible phlebotomy practice. By recognizing the signs of complications early and implementing appropriate corrective measures, phlebotomists can navigate challenging situations while minimizing potential patient risks.

Common Complications and Troubleshooting:

1. **Hematoma Formation:**
   - **Cause:** A hematoma forms when blood leaks into the surrounding tissue due to improper needle insertion or accidental needle movement within the vein. This can also happen if the tourniquet is too close to the site.
   - **Troubleshooting:** If a hematoma forms, immediately release the tourniquet, stop blood collection, and gently remove the needle. Apply pressure with sterile gauze to minimize bleeding and promote clotting. Advise the patient to keep the area elevated and apply cold compresses to reduce swelling.
2. **Infiltration:**
   - **Cause:** Infiltration occurs when fluid from the intravenous line enters the surrounding tissue due to the needle dislodging from the vein.
   - **Troubleshooting:** If infiltration is suspected, stop blood collection, remove the needle, and apply

pressure with sterile gauze to reduce swelling. Elevate the affected limb and encourage movement to disperse the fluid. Document the incident and inform the healthcare team if necessary.

3. **Venous Spasm:**
   - **Cause:** Venous spasm is an involuntary vein contraction, often in response to discomfort, anxiety, or a sudden movement.
   - **Troubleshooting:** If venous spasm occurs, gently massage the affected area to help relax the vein. If the spasm persists, consider reattempting venipuncture at a different site. Prioritize patient comfort and communication throughout the process.

4. **Partial Tube Filling:**
   - **Cause:** Tubes may not fill adequately if the needle is not correctly positioned within the vein or if the tube is not securely attached.
   - **Troubleshooting:** If a tube is only partially filled, ensure the needle is correctly placed within the vein. Confirm that the tube is securely attached to the needle and reattempt blood collection if necessary.

5. **Patient Fainting or Vasovagal Response:**
   - **Cause:** Some patients may experience fainting, dizziness, or a vasovagal response due to anxiety or fear of needles. (AKA Syncope)
   - **Troubleshooting:** If a patient exhibits these

symptoms, immediately stop the procedure, safely remove the needle, and assist the patient into a reclined position. Provide a cold compress and reassurance. Monitor the patient until they feel stable and are ready to leave.

Prevention and Mitigation:

- **Proper Technique:** Use proper needle insertion technique, stabilization, and patient positioning to minimize the risk of complications.
- **Communication:** Maintain open communication with patients to address their concerns, fears, and any discomfort they experience.
- **Patient Education:** Inform patients about potential complications and reassure them that prompt action will be taken if any arise.

Conclusion: Complications can challenge even the most skilled phlebotomists. By understanding the causes, recognizing the signs, and employing effective troubleshooting strategies, phlebotomists demonstrate their commitment to patient safety and optimal blood collection outcomes. Rapid and decisive response to complications reflects the dedication of phlebotomists to ensuring a safe and positive patient experience.

3. Special Populations and Considerations

Phlebotomists encounter diverse patients, each with unique needs and considerations. Special populations, including pediatric, geriatric, and patients with specific medical conditions, require tailored approaches to blood collection procedures. This section delves into the techniques, strategies, and considerations that phlebotomists should employ when working with special populations, ensuring their safety, comfort, and overall well-being. Recognizing special populations' distinct characteristics and requirements is essential for personalized and compassionate care. Whether dealing with the vulnerability of pediatric patients, the complexities of geriatric patients, or the challenges posed by patients with medical conditions, phlebotomists play a crucial role in adapting their approach to ensure successful blood collection.

Pediatric Patients:

1. **Communication:** Use child-friendly language to explain the procedure, involving caregivers and offering reassurance.
2. **Distraction Techniques:** Employ distraction techniques, such as toys, games, or colorful visuals, to ease anxiety and redirect focus.
3. **Engagement:** Ask pediatric patients about their preferences, such as which arm they would like to use or if they have any comfort items.
4. **Gentle Touch:** Use a gentle touch and avoid sudden movements to prevent startling the child.

Geriatric Patients:

1. **Respectful Communication:** Speak clearly and respectfully to elderly patients, allowing them ample time to process information and ask questions.
2. **Comfortable Positioning:** Ensure comfortable positioning, supporting mobility limitations or physical discomfort.
3. **Clear Explanation:** Offer a clear and concise explanation of the procedure, addressing concerns and accommodating hearing or visual impairments.
4. **Patience:** Demonstrate patience and understanding, allowing extra time for the patient to follow instructions and cooperate.
5.

Patients with Medical Conditions:

1. **Chronic Illnesses:** Be aware of chronic illnesses, medications, and potential blood collection complications.
2. **Allergies:** Ask about allergies or sensitivities to adhesive materials, antiseptics, or latex to prevent adverse reactions.
3. **Blood Disorders:** Exercise caution when working with patients with bleeding disorders, adjusting techniques to minimize bruising or complications.
4. **Fasting Patients:** For patients requiring fasting blood work, ensure they are well-informed about fasting requirements and schedule appointments accordingly.

Bariatric Patients:

1. **Vein Selection:** Carefully select a suitable vein, considering the patient's body composition and vein accessibility.
2. **Tourniquet Application:** Apply the tourniquet firmly but cautiously to avoid causing discomfort or harm.
3. **Needle Insertion:** Use an appropriate needle length and angle to accommodate the patient's body size.

Cultural Sensitivity:

1. **Language Barriers:** Use interpreters or translation services to bridge language gaps and ensure accurate communication.
2. **Cultural Practices:** Respect patients' cultural practices, sensitivities, and preferences, adapting the approach accordingly.

Conclusion: Working with special populations demands heightened sensitivity, adaptability, and skill. By tailoring approaches, employing specialized techniques, and fostering an environment of trust and respect, phlebotomists ensure that blood collection procedures are safe, effective, and comfortable for every patient. The ability to navigate the unique needs of special populations underscores the commitment of phlebotomists to providing patient-centered care that upholds the principles of compassion, diversity, and inclusion.

Pediatric Phlebotomy Techniques

Phlebotomy procedures for pediatric patients require unique skills, considerations, and approaches. Children's reactions to medical procedures can range from curiosity to fear, making it essential for phlebotomists to be adept at creating a supportive and reassuring environment. "Pediatric Phlebotomy Techniques" is a specialized field focusing on blood collection from infants, toddlers, children, and adolescents. In this section, we explore the intricacies of pediatric phlebotomy, emphasizing the importance of gentle techniques, effective communication, and age-appropriate strategies to ensure successful blood collection while prioritizing the well-being of young patients.

Understanding pediatric patients' distinct physical, emotional, and psychological needs is paramount. Successful pediatric phlebotomy requires technical proficiency, an understanding of child development, effective communication, and the ability to address the anxieties of both the child and their caregivers.

This section will explore various aspects of pediatric phlebotomy techniques. From selecting appropriate venipuncture sites and implementing distraction techniques to tailoring communication to children's understanding, we aim to equip phlebotomists with the tools to create positive experiences for young patients. By demonstrating empathy, patience, and expertise, phlebotomists contribute to reducing the stress and anxiety associated with medical procedures for children and their families.

Ultimately, mastering pediatric phlebotomy techniques underscores the commitment of phlebotomists to delivering safe, compassionate, and patient-centered care. As we delve into the strategies and considerations specific to pediatric blood collection, we aim to empower phlebotomists to be effective advocates for the health and comfort of the youngest members of our community.

Age-Appropriate Communication:

1. **Visual Aids:** Utilize visual aids such as pictures, diagrams, or cartoons to explain the procedure in a child-friendly manner.
2. **Child-Centered Language:** Avoid medical jargon and use age-appropriate language and explanations children can understand.
3. **Engage the Child:** Involve the child in decision-making, such as selecting the arm for venipuncture, to provide a sense of control.
4. **Reassurance:** Offer consistent reassurance that the procedure will be brief and comfortable. Let them know that they will only feel a slight pinch. Never say to them that they will not feel a thing.

Distraction Techniques:

1. **Toys and Distractions:** Provide toys, bubbles, or handheld electronic devices to divert the child's attention during the procedure.

2. **Storytelling:** Narrate a story or engage the child in conversation to distract from the procedure.

3. **Singing or Counting:** Sing a familiar song or engage the child in counting, providing a pleasant distraction.

Age-Specific Techniques:

1. **Infants and Toddlers:** Opt for heels or the lateral plantar surface for capillary blood collection. Use a pacifier dipped in a sweet solution to soothe infants during the procedure.

2. **Preschoolers:** Offer choices, such as selecting the hand for venipuncture, to empower children and provide a sense of control.

3. **School-age children:** Explain the procedure using simple terms, allowing them to ask questions and voice concerns.

4. **Adolescents:** Respect their need for privacy and provide information about the procedure's purpose and importance.

Vein Selection:

1. **Hand Veins:** Hand veins are often more visible and accessible in children. Consider them for venipuncture if appropriate.

2. **Distal Sites:** Opt for veins in distal areas, as they are generally less painful and offer a better chance of success.

Minimizing Discomfort:

1. **Topical Anesthetics:** Consider using a topical anesthetic cream to numb the skin before venipuncture.
2. **Warm Compress:** Apply a warm compress to enhance vein visibility and comfort.

Conclusion:

Pediatric phlebotomy techniques encompass a blend of technical skills and compassionate care. By employing age-appropriate communication, distraction techniques, and specialized approaches for different age groups, phlebotomists create a positive experience for young patients and their families. Adapting and connecting with children ensures successful blood collection procedures while nurturing a sense of trust and confidence in the healthcare environment. Pediatric phlebotomy techniques reflect the dedication of phlebotomists to the principles of patient-centered care, compassion, and excellence in their practice.

Geriatric Phlebotomy Techniques

Geriatric patients in the advanced stages of life present distinct considerations and challenges regarding phlebotomy procedures. As the aging population continues to grow, phlebotomists must be well-versed in addressing the unique needs and sensitivities of elderly individuals during blood collection. This section explores the specialized techniques and considerations involved in performing phlebotomy on geriatric patients, ensuring their comfort, safety, and overall well-being.

Geriatric phlebotomy requires an approach that considers the physiological changes, medical conditions, and potential vulnerabilities of aging. Geriatric patients often have fragile skin, reduced vein elasticity, and a higher likelihood of chronic illnesses. As a result, phlebotomists must adopt strategies that prioritize patient comfort, minimize complications, and promote optimal blood collection outcomes.

Considerations for Geriatric Phlebotomy:
1. **Vein Fragility:** Elderly patients often have fragile veins prone to bruising and damage. Choose vein sites carefully and use gentle techniques to minimize trauma.
2. **Venipuncture Sites:** Opt for easily accessible veins in areas such as the forearm or hand. Avoid using veins over bony prominences to prevent discomfort.

3. **Communication:** Speak clearly and respectfully to elderly patients, allowing them ample time to process information and ask questions.
4. **Comfortable Positioning:** Ensure elderly patients are positioned comfortably, considering mobility limitations or physical discomfort.
5. **Tourniquet Application:** Apply the tourniquet cautiously, avoiding excessive pressure that may cause discomfort or harm.
6. **Needle Size and Angle:** Select an appropriate needle size and angle that accommodate the patient's vein condition and body composition.
7. **Patient Dignity:** Respect patient dignity by providing privacy, covering them appropriately, and maintaining a warm environment.
8. **Pain Management:** Prioritize pain management by using distraction techniques, providing reassurance, and using appropriate local anesthesia if necessary.
9. **Slow Blood Collection:** Geriatric patients may require slower blood collection to prevent adverse reactions or discomfort.
10. **Caregiver Involvement:** Involve caregivers or family members as necessary to provide emotional support and ensure the patient's well-being.

Benefits of Geriatric Phlebotomy Considerations:

- **Patient Comfort:** By addressing the unique needs of geriatric patients, phlebotomists enhance patient comfort during blood collection procedures.
- **Minimized Complications:** Employing specialized techniques reduces the risk of complications such as bruising, hematoma formation, or vein damage.
- **Patient-Centered Care:** Geriatric phlebotomy practices align with patient-centered care principles, emphasizing respect and individualized attention.

Conclusion:

Geriatric phlebotomy considerations reflect the commitment of phlebotomists to providing safe, compassionate, and personalized care to the elderly population. By tailoring techniques to the specific needs of geriatric patients, phlebotomists contribute to positive patient experiences and uphold the principles of dignity, respect, and excellence in healthcare. Geriatric phlebotomy is not only a technical skill but also an expression of the dedication to improving the well-being of patients in their later years.

1. Phlebotomy for Patients with Difficult Veins

Patients with problematic veins present a unique challenge to phlebotomists, as their veins may be less visible, palpable, or prone to collapsing during blood collection procedures. Successfully obtaining blood samples from these patients requires specialized techniques, adaptability, and a thorough understanding of vein anatomy and behavior. This section explores the strategies and considerations involved in performing phlebotomy on patients with difficult veins, ensuring accurate sample collection while prioritizing patient comfort and safety.

Patients with difficult veins pose a distinct challenge due to obesity, dehydration, scar tissue, or medical conditions that affect vein visibility and accessibility. Overcoming these challenges requires phlebotomists to adopt innovative approaches that optimize the chances of successful venipuncture while minimizing patient discomfort and the risk of complications.

Strategies for Phlebotomy on Patients with Difficult Veins:

1. **Vein Selection Expertise:** Utilize advanced palpation techniques to locate veins that may not be immediately visible.
2. **Use of Warm Compresses:** Apply warm compresses to dilate veins and enhance visibility, especially in patients with constricted veins.
3. **Gravity-Assisted Techniques:** Position the patient's arm downward to encourage blood flow to the veins, making them more accessible.
4. **Blood Pressure Cuff Technique:** Apply a blood pressure cuff to create a controlled tourniquet effect, aiding vein engorgement.

5. **Distal Vein Selection:** Choose veins in distal areas, such as the hand, fingers, or wrist, which may be more visible and accessible.

6. **Utilize Transillumination:** A transilluminator will illuminate veins underneath the skin, enhancing their visibility.

7. **Ultrasound Guidance:** In challenging cases, consider ultrasound guidance to locate veins for successful venipuncture accurately.

8. **Hydration Promotion:** Encourage patients to hydrate adequately before blood collection to improve vein pliability and visibility.

9. **Accurate Needle Insertion:** Use a slow and controlled needle insertion technique to prevent vein collapse.

Considerations for Patients with Difficult Veins:

- **Patient Communication:** Inform patients about the challenges of difficult veins, set appropriate expectations, and reassure them that efforts will be made to minimize discomfort.

- **Needle Gauge Selection:** Choose a slightly larger needle gauge, like 23g, to increase the chances of successful venipuncture.

- **Collaboration:** Collaborate with colleagues, supervisors, or other healthcare professionals when faced with particularly challenging cases.

Benefits of Phlebotomy Techniques for Difficult Veins:

- **Successful Collection:** Effective strategies enhance the chances of obtaining accurate blood samples from patients with difficult veins.

- **Reduced Discomfort:** Specialized techniques minimize patient discomfort by optimizing the chances of a single successful venipuncture.

- **Patient Satisfaction:** By adapting to patients with difficult veins' unique needs, phlebotomists contribute to positive patient experiences.

Conclusion:

Phlebotomy for patients with difficult veins requires skill, innovation, and adaptability. Phlebotomists can overcome challenges and ensure successful blood collection by applying advanced techniques and utilizing specialized tools. The ability to perform phlebotomy on patients with difficult veins demonstrates the commitment of phlebotomists to patient-centered care, accuracy, and excellence in their practice.

Blood Collection in Emergency Situations

Emergencies often require swift and accurate blood collection to aid diagnosis, treatment, and patient management. Phlebotomists play a critical role in these scenarios by quickly and efficiently obtaining blood samples while prioritizing patient safety and adhering to established protocols. This section explores the specialized techniques, considerations, and strategies for blood collection in emergencies, ensuring timely and reliable sample acquisition to support urgent medical care.

In emergencies, time is of the essence, and phlebotomists must be prepared to collect blood samples rapidly and effectively. These situations may arise in emergency departments, trauma centers, critical care units, or during pre-hospital care. Performing blood collection under pressure while maintaining accuracy and adhering to safety protocols is crucial to delivering optimal patient care.

Strategies for Blood Collection in Emergency Situations:
1. **Preparation:** Ensure necessary equipment, supplies, and labeling materials are readily available.
2. **Team Collaboration:** Communicate effectively with other healthcare team members to ensure coordinated care and minimal disruption.
3. **Patient Stabilization:** Prioritize patient stabilization and safety before initiating blood collection procedures.

4. **Rapid Identification:** Confirm patient identification using two unique identifiers to prevent errors.

5. **Minimal Disruption:** Perform blood collection quickly and efficiently to minimize patient discomfort and disruption to ongoing care.

6. **Proper Needle Insertion:** Maintain focus on proper needle insertion technique to ensure accuracy and reduce the risk of complications.

7. **Safe Disposal:** Properly dispose of sharps and biohazardous waste in accordance with established guidelines.

8. **Documentation:** Accurately document all procedures, including the date, time, patient information, and the person who collected the sample.

Considerations for Blood Collection in Emergency Situations:

- **Patient Prioritization:** Assess the patient's condition and stability before initiating blood collection, and communicate with the healthcare team if priorities change.

- **Minimal Blood Volume:** Collect the minimum volume required for urgent tests to conserve blood and minimize patient stress.

- **Patient Comfort:** Despite the urgency, prioritize patient comfort and reassurance during the blood collection.

Benefits of Blood Collection Techniques in Emergency Situations:

- **Urgent Diagnosis:** Timely blood collection enables rapid diagnosis and treatment decisions in critical situations.
- **Effective Patient Management:** Accurate blood test results support appropriate medical interventions and patient management.
- **Collaborative Care:** Coordinated blood collection enhances communication and collaboration among healthcare team members.

Conclusion:

Blood collection in emergency situations demands unique skills, adaptability, and a commitment to patient-centered care. Phlebotomists proficient in collecting blood samples swiftly and accurately under pressure contribute significantly to the timely delivery of medical care in critical moments. By prioritizing patient safety, efficient techniques, and seamless collaboration with the healthcare team, phlebotomists play a vital role in supporting emergency medical interventions and ensuring the best possible outcomes for patients facing urgent medical challenges.

Handling and Labeling Collected Specimens

Once blood samples are successfully collected, proper handling and accurate labeling of specimens are critical to maintaining the integrity of diagnostic testing and ensuring patient safety. Phlebotomists play a pivotal role in this stage of the process, as errors or mishandling can lead to inaccurate results, misdiagnosis, or treatment complications. This section examines the essential practices and considerations for handling and labeling collected specimens, highlighting the importance of meticulous attention to detail, adherence to protocols, and safeguarding patient information. Proper specimen handling and labeling not only contribute to the accuracy of laboratory tests but also reflect the commitment of phlebotomists to maintaining the highest standards of patient care and ensuring that healthcare professionals receive reliable information for clinical decision-making.

Throughout this section, we explore the precise techniques for correctly handling blood specimens, proper storage methods, and the importance of accurate and legible labeling. As we delve into these aspects, phlebotomists will gain insights into their pivotal role in preserving the quality and reliability of specimens, ultimately upholding the principles of patient safety, accuracy, and excellence in laboratory practices.

1. Centrifugation and Serum/Plasma Separation

After collecting blood specimens, they often need to be processed to separate the serum or plasma from the cellular components. This separation is crucial for accurate diagnostic testing, as it allows for analyzing specific components without interference from other blood elements. In this section, we explore the process of centrifugation, which plays a pivotal role in separating serum or plasma from whole blood, and the subsequent handling of these components.

Centrifugation is a vital step in the laboratory workflow that separates blood into its constituent parts based on density. This process is essential for creating clear serum or plasma samples for testing, free from cellular elements that could affect the results. Proper centrifugation techniques ensure the separated serum or plasma can be accurately analyzed, leading to reliable diagnostic information.

Centrifugation Process:

1. **Equipment Preparation:** Ensure the centrifuge is calibrated correctly, balanced, and loaded with the appropriate specimens.
2. **Tube Identification:** Clearly label tubes with patient information and specimen details to prevent mix-ups during centrifugation.
3. **Centrifuge Settings:** Set the centrifuge to the appropriate speed and duration based on the laboratory's protocols and

the type of test to be performed.

4. **Balancing:** Place an equal number of tubes on opposite sides of the centrifuge rotor to maintain balance and prevent vibration.

5. **Centrifugation:** Activate the centrifuge and allow it to reach the desired speed. The centrifugal force will cause the denser cellular elements to settle at the bottom, while the serum or plasma will rise to the top.

6. **Deceleration:** Once centrifugation is complete, gradually decelerate the rotor to avoid disturbing the separated layers.

Serum/Plasma Separation:

1. **Extraction:** Using a pipette or other appropriate tool, carefully extract the serum or plasma from the top layer without disturbing the cellular components below.

2. **Transfer:** Transfer the extracted serum or plasma into labeled collection tubes for testing, ensuring accurate and legible labeling.

3. **Avoid Hemolysis:** Exercise caution to prevent hemolysis (rupturing of red blood cells) during the separation process, as it can affect test results.

Considerations for Centrifugation and Serum/Plasma Separation:

- **Time and Speed:** Adhere to established centrifugation parameters to ensure consistent results and prevent sample degradation.

- **Labeling:** Properly label tubes with patient information, test details, and collection date and time to prevent errors.
- **Serum vs. Plasma:** Be aware of the specific requirements for each test. Some tests require serum, while others require plasma, which necessitates using appropriate collection tubes.
- **Gentle Handling:** Handle extracted serum or plasma gently to avoid contamination or hemolysis, which can affect test accuracy.

Benefits of Proper Centrifugation and Separation:

- **Accurate Results:** Proper centrifugation and separation techniques lead to clear, uncontaminated serum or plasma samples, ensuring accurate diagnostic results.
- **Minimal Interference:** Separating cellular elements from serum or plasma minimizes interference in laboratory testing, yielding reliable data.
- **Patient Safety:** Accurate test results contribute to safe and effective patient management and treatment decisions.

Conclusion:

Centrifugation and serum/plasma separation are critical steps in the laboratory process that demand meticulous attention to detail. Phlebotomists who execute these techniques ensure that diagnostic testing is based on accurate and uncontaminated samples, reflecting their dedication to patient care and the highest laboratory practice standards. Proper centrifugation and separation techniques contribute to laboratory results' accuracy and reliability, supporting healthcare professionals in delivering optimal patient care.

2. Proper Storage and Transport of Specimens

Once blood specimens are collected, processed, and separated, their proper storage and transportation are vital to maintaining sample integrity and ensuring accurate laboratory results. Phlebotomists are crucial in ensuring that specimens are handled, stored, and transported according to established protocols and guidelines. This section delves into the essential practices for properly storing and transporting specimens, emphasizing temperature control, protection from contamination, and adherence to regulatory standards.

Proper storage and transport of specimens are integral components of maintaining the quality of blood samples and upholding the accuracy of laboratory testing. Handling specimens beyond collection involves safeguarding against factors that could compromise the integrity of samples, such as temperature fluctuations, contamination, and mishandling. Phlebotomists' attention to detail and adherence to established protocols contribute significantly to the reliability of test results and the overall delivery of patient care.

Considerations for Proper Storage and Transport:

1. **Temperature Control:**
   - Maintain specimens at appropriate temperatures based on test requirements. Refrigerate or freeze specimens as needed to prevent degradation.
   - Monitor temperature storage conditions using temperature logs, monitoring devices, or temperature-controlled storage units.

2. **Protection from Contamination:**
   - Store specimens in leak-proof, airtight containers to prevent cross-contamination and maintain sample integrity.
   - Ensure proper labeling of containers to avoid mix-ups and confusion.

3. **Timely Transport:**
   - Transport specimens to the laboratory promptly after collection and processing to prevent degradation or alteration of samples.

4. **Packaging Guidelines:**
   - Use secure packaging that provides cushioning and protection to prevent breakage or leakage during transportation.

5. **Transportation Compliance:**
   - Adhere to transportation regulations, including those outlined by regulatory bodies and transport companies, to ensure legal and safe transport.

6. **Chain of Custody:**
   - Maintain a clear chain of custody record, documenting the movement and handling of specimens to ensure traceability and accountability.

7. **Patient Privacy:**
   - Protect patient confidentiality by appropriately labeling and securely packaging specimens during transport.

8. **Emergency Procedures:**
   - Establish procedures for handling unexpected delays, adverse weather conditions, or transport disruptions to prevent sample compromise.

Benefits of Proper Storage and Transport:

- **Accurate Results:** Proper storage and transport help maintain the integrity of samples, leading to accurate and reliable laboratory results.

- **Regulatory Compliance:** Adhering to storage and transport guidelines ensures compliance with regulatory standards and best practices.

- **Patient Care:** Reliable test results support accurate diagnosis and appropriate patient management, contributing to effective healthcare delivery.

Conclusion:

Proper storage and transport of specimens are integral aspects of phlebotomy practice that demand meticulous attention and adherence to guidelines. By safeguarding specimens against temperature fluctuations, contamination, and mishandling, phlebotomists play a critical role in maintaining sample integrity and preserving the accuracy of laboratory testing. Demonstrating competence in proper storage and transport techniques reflects the dedication of phlebotomists to patient safety, data accuracy, and the highest standards of laboratory practices.

3. Chain of Custody and Specimen Integrity

Maintaining the chain of custody and ensuring specimen integrity is fundamental to preserving laboratory test results' reliability and legal validity. The chain of custody refers to the documented trail that tracks a specimen's handling, storage, and transport from the point of collection to the laboratory analysis. In this section, we explore the significance of maintaining a robust chain of custody, the steps involved, and the practices that ensure specimen integrity throughout the process.

The chain of custody is a critical component of specimen handling that ensures each specimen's accountability, traceability, and authenticity as it moves through various stages of the testing process. A well-maintained chain of custody helps prevent contamination, tampering, or mishandling, which could compromise the validity of test results and legal proceedings that may involve the specimens.

Maintaining the Chain of Custody:
1. **Proper Labeling:** Accurately label specimens with patient information, collection date and time, and other necessary details.
2. **Documentation:** Document every transfer or change in custody with signatures, dates, times, and details of individuals involved.
3. **Secure Packaging:** Store and transport specimens in secure, sealed containers to prevent unauthorized access or tampering.
4. **Record Keeping:** Maintain comprehensive records of the chain of custody, including names, signatures, and timestamps.
5. **Digital Documentation:** Utilize electronic systems for documenting the chain of custody, ensuring accurate and accessible records.
6. **Security Measures:** Implement security protocols, such as locked storage areas and access controls, to prevent unauthorized handling.
7. **Transport Monitoring:** Monitor and document the temperature and conditions during specimen transportation to ensure stability.

Ensuring Specimen Integrity:

1. **Proper Handling:** Handle specimens carefully to prevent contamination or degradation during collection, processing, and transport.

2. **Temperature Control:** Maintain proper temperature conditions to prevent degradation and maintain sample stability.

3. **Sealed Containers:** Store specimens in sealed containers to prevent leakage and maintain sample integrity.

4. **Avoid Cross-Contamination:** Adhere to sterile techniques and prevent cross-contamination to ensure accurate test results.

5. **Label Accuracy:** To prevent mix-ups, verify and confirm specimen labeling accuracy at each transfer point.

6. **Secure Storage:** Store specimens in designated, secure areas to prevent unauthorized access and ensure sample integrity.

Benefits of Chain of Custody and Specimen Integrity:

- **Legal Validity:** A well-documented chain of custody enhances the legal validity of test results in court proceedings or legal disputes.

- **Reliable Results:** Specimen integrity ensures that test results accurately reflect the patient's condition and are contamination-free.

- **Professional Accountability:** Demonstrating adherence to the chain of custody protocols reflects professionalism, responsibility, and commitment to accurate practices.

Conclusion:

Maintaining the chain of custody and ensuring specimen integrity are foundational to reliable laboratory testing. Phlebotomists' diligence in accurately documenting every step of the process and safeguarding specimens against contamination or tampering contributes to test results' accuracy, legality, and credibility. By prioritizing the chain of custody and specimen integrity, phlebotomists play a vital role in upholding patient safety, healthcare quality, and the integrity of laboratory practices.

Introduction to Laboratory Testing

Laboratory testing is a cornerstone of modern healthcare, providing valuable insights into a patient's health, diagnosing diseases, monitoring treatment progress, and guiding medical decisions. Collecting high-quality blood samples is the first step toward generating accurate and reliable laboratory results within phlebotomy. This section delves into the essential principles of laboratory testing, the various types of tests conducted, and the critical role that phlebotomists play in ensuring the integrity of specimens for accurate analysis.

Laboratory testing involves the examination of various bodily substances, including blood, urine, and tissues, to gather information about a patient's health status. These tests provide clinicians with objective data that aid in diagnosing conditions, determining appropriate treatments, and evaluating the effectiveness of interventions. Accurate laboratory results are crucial for delivering effective and personalized patient care, enhancing patient outcomes, and guiding medical decision-making.

Types of Laboratory Tests:

1. **Diagnostic Tests:** These tests identify the presence or absence of a disease or condition, aiding in the initial diagnosis. Examples include blood glucose tests for diabetes and complete blood counts (CBC) to assess overall health.

2. **Monitoring Tests:** Monitoring tests track the progression of a disease, the impact of treatments, or the effects of medications. Examples include measuring cholesterol levels in patients on lipid-lowering medications.
3. **Screening Tests:** Screening tests identify potential health issues in asymptomatic individuals. Examples include cancer screenings such as mammograms and PSA tests.
4. **Prognostic Tests:** Prognostic tests provide information about the likely course of a disease, helping healthcare providers anticipate potential outcomes and tailor treatment plans accordingly.
5. **Genetic Tests:** Genetic tests analyze an individual's DNA to identify genetic predispositions to diseases or determine appropriate treatments.

1. Phlebotomists' Role in Laboratory Testing:

Phlebotomists are integral to the laboratory testing process as they collect blood samples accurately and safely. Their expertise in venipuncture, specimen handling, and protocol adherence directly impact the quality of laboratory results. Phlebotomists' attention to detail, patient-centered care, and adherence to established practices contribute to reliable and accurate laboratory testing outcomes.

Impact on Patient Care:

Reliable laboratory results obtained through meticulous phlebotomy and proper specimen handling directly influence patient care in the following ways:

- **Accurate Diagnoses:** Precise laboratory results enable healthcare providers to diagnose conditions and tailor treatment plans accurately.

- **Effective Treatment:** Lab tests guide the choice and adjustment of treatments, ensuring that interventions are appropriate and effective.

- **Early Detection:** Screening tests can detect conditions in their early stages, allowing for timely interventions and improved outcomes.

- **Progress Monitoring:** Regular laboratory testing helps clinicians monitor disease progression and treatment efficacy.

- **Preventive Measures:** Genetic tests offer insights into risk factors, enabling individuals to make informed decisions about preventive measures.

Conclusion:

Laboratory testing is a cornerstone of evidence-based medicine, and phlebotomists' role in collecting high-quality blood samples is pivotal to the accuracy and reliability of these tests. By adhering to best practices, prioritizing patient comfort and safety, and maintaining specimen integrity, phlebotomists contribute significantly to generating accurate and actionable laboratory results. These results, in turn, empower healthcare professionals to provide optimal patient care, patient outcomes, and medical decisions.

2. Standard Blood Tests and Their Significance

Standard routine or basic blood tests are fundamental diagnostic tools that provide essential information about a patient's overall health, organ function, and potential health risks. These tests encompass a range of measurements that offer insights into various aspects of the body's physiological processes. In this section, we delve into the significance of standard blood tests, the specific parameters they assess, and their role in guiding medical decision-making.

Standard blood tests form the foundation of laboratory diagnostics, allowing healthcare providers to assess a patient's health status and identify potential underlying issues. These tests are routinely performed during wellness check-ups, medical evaluations, and disease management to gather objective data that support clinical assessments and treatment decisions.

Common Parameters Assessed in Standard Blood Tests:

1. **Complete Blood Count (CBC):** A CBC provides information about the blood composition, including red and white blood cell counts, hemoglobin levels, and platelet counts. It helps diagnose anemia, infections, and various blood disorders.

2. **Basic Metabolic Panel (BMP):** The BMP measures electrolytes, glucose, and kidney function indicators like creatinine and blood urea nitrogen (BUN). It aids in assessing

kidney function, electrolyte balance, and blood sugar levels.

3. **Comprehensive Metabolic Panel (CMP):** Similar to the BMP, the CMP includes additional liver function tests, such as liver enzymes and bilirubin levels, providing insights into liver health and metabolism.

4. **Lipid Panel:** The lipid panel measures cholesterol levels, triglycerides, high-density lipoprotein (HDL), and low-density lipoprotein (LDL) cholesterol. It assesses cardiovascular health and the risk of heart disease.

5. **Thyroid Function Tests:** These tests, including TSH (thyroid-stimulating hormone), T3 (triiodothyronine), and T4 (thyroxine), evaluate thyroid gland function and hormone levels.

6. **Blood Glucose Test:** The blood glucose test measures the amount of sugar in the blood, assisting in diagnosing and monitoring diabetes and metabolic disorders.

Significance of Standard Blood Tests:

1. **Early Detection:** Routine blood tests can detect health issues in their early stages, allowing for timely interventions and preventive measures.

2. **Health Monitoring:** Regular blood tests help healthcare providers monitor disease progression, treatment effectiveness, and overall health status.

3. **Risk Assessment:** Blood tests provide insights into risk factors for various conditions, enabling individuals to make

informed lifestyle changes.

4. **Treatment Decision-Making:** Test results guide treatment choices and adjustments, ensuring personalized and effective patient care.

5. **Baseline Information:** Blood tests establish baseline health information for future comparisons, aiding in assessing health trends over time.

Conclusion:

Standard blood tests are foundational in healthcare, offering valuable insights into a patient's health, identifying potential issues, and guiding medical decisions. By assessing a range of parameters related to blood composition, organ function, and metabolic processes, these tests empower healthcare providers to diagnose conditions, monitor health, and tailor interventions. Phlebotomists contribute to the reliability and accuracy of these tests by skillfully collecting blood samples, ensuring proper handling, and maintaining specimen integrity, ultimately supporting optimal patient care.

3. Hematology, Chemistry, and Microbiology Tests

Hematology, chemistry, and microbiology tests encompass diverse laboratory analyses that delve deeper into specific aspects of a patient's health. These specialized tests provide valuable insights into blood disorders, organ function, and infectious diseases. This section explores the significance of hematology, chemistry, and microbiology tests, the parameters they assess, and their role in enhancing medical diagnoses and treatment strategies.

Hematology tests focus on the cellular and molecular components of blood, chemistry tests analyze blood chemistry and organ function, and microbiology tests identify infectious agents. Together, these tests offer comprehensive information about a patient's health and aid in diagnosing various medical conditions.

Hematology Tests and Their Significance:
1. **Coagulation Tests:** Coagulation tests assess blood clotting function, helping diagnose clotting disorders like hemophilia and monitoring anticoagulant therapy.
2. **Peripheral Blood Smear:** This test examines blood cells under a microscope, identifying red and white blood cell abnormalities.
3. **Hematocrit and Hemoglobin:** These tests measure blood volume and oxygen-carrying capacity, aiding in diagnosing anemia and monitoring blood loss.
4. **Platelet Count:** Platelet count assesses clotting function and identifies disorders like thrombocytopenia or thrombocytosis.

Chemistry Tests and Their Significance:
1. **Liver Function Tests:** These tests evaluate liver health by measuring enzymes, bilirubin, and proteins. They aid in diagnosing liver diseases and monitoring liver function.

2. **Kidney Function Tests:** Kidney function tests assess creatinine, BUN, and electrolyte levels, aiding in diagnosing kidney diseases and evaluating kidney health.

3. **Electrolyte Panel:** Electrolyte tests measure essential minerals like sodium, potassium, and calcium, providing insights into fluid balance and overall health.

4. **Glucose Tolerance Test:** This test assesses how the body processes glucose and helps diagnose diabetes and insulin resistance.

Microbiology Tests and Their Significance:

1. **Cultures:** Microbial cultures identify and isolate infectious agents, helping diagnose bacterial, viral, or fungal infections.

2. **Sensitivity Testing:** Sensitivity tests determine the most effective antibiotics to treat specific infections, guiding antibiotic therapy.

3. **Molecular Testing:** Molecular tests detect DNA or RNA of pathogens, providing rapid and accurate identification of infectious agents.

Significance of Hematology, Chemistry, and Microbiology Tests:

1. **Precise Diagnoses:** Specialized tests provide specific information about blood, organ function, and pathogens, aiding in precise diagnoses.

2. **Tailored Treatment:** Test results guide personalized treatment strategies, optimizing therapy effectiveness and

minimizing adverse effects.

3. **Infection Control:** Microbiology tests aid in identifying infectious agents, enabling timely treatment and infection control measures.

4. **Disease Monitoring:** Hematology and chemistry tests assist in monitoring disease progression, treatment efficacy, and patient recovery.

Conclusion:

Hematology, chemistry, and microbiology tests expand the diagnostic capabilities of healthcare professionals, offering detailed insights into specific aspects of a patient's health. These tests are vital in diagnosing blood disorders, evaluating organ function, and identifying infectious agents. By conducting these tests accurately, phlebotomists contribute to the accuracy and reliability of diagnostic results, ultimately enhancing patient care, treatment outcomes, and disease management strategies.

4. Quality Assurance and Error Prevention

Maintaining the highest quality assurance standards and implementing robust error prevention measures are essential in laboratory testing. Accuracy, reliability, and patient safety depend on the diligent efforts of healthcare professionals, including phlebotomists, who collect and handle specimens. This section looks into the significance of quality assurance, error prevention principles, and phlebotomists' role in upholding these practices.

Quality assurance involves systematic measures to ensure that laboratory processes consistently produce accurate and reliable results. Error prevention focuses on identifying potential sources of mistakes and implementing safeguards to mitigate their impact. Adhering to stringent quality assurance practices and error prevention strategies in phlebotomy is paramount to delivering safe and precise laboratory testing outcomes.

Principles of Quality Assurance:

1. **Standardization:** Establish standardized procedures for specimen collection, handling, processing, and testing to minimize variability.
2. **Training and Competency:** Ensure phlebotomists are well-trained, competent, and continually updated on best practices and protocols.
3. **Documentation:** Maintain comprehensive records of procedures, instrument maintenance, and personnel qualifications.
4. **Instrument Calibration:** Regularly calibrate and maintain laboratory equipment to ensure accurate and consistent results.
5. **Proficiency Testing:** Participate in external proficiency testing programs to verify the accuracy of laboratory testing procedures.

Error Prevention Strategies:

1. **Double-Check Procedures:** Implement a two-person verification process for critical steps, such as patient identification and labeling.

2. **Barcode Scanning:** Utilize barcode scanning technology to ensure accurate patient identification and specimen tracking.

3. **Specimen Labeling:** Prioritize accurate and legible specimen labeling, adhering to best practices for patient identification.

4. **Documentation Review:** Review all documentation, including requisitions and orders, to ensure accuracy before proceeding with procedures.

5. **Communication:** Maintain clear and open communication among healthcare team members to prevent misunderstandings and errors.

Role of Phlebotomists in Quality Assurance:

Phlebotomists are at the forefront of specimen collection and handling, making their role crucial in maintaining quality assurance and preventing errors. Their adherence to protocols, attention to detail, and commitment to patient safety contribute to accurate and reliable laboratory results.

Benefits of Quality Assurance and Error Prevention:

1. **Patient Safety:** Rigorous quality assurance practices prevent errors that could harm patients or lead to misdiagnosis.

2. **Reliability:** Ensuring the accuracy and reliability of test

results instills confidence in healthcare providers' decisions.

3. **Regulatory Compliance:** Adhering to quality assurance standards ensures compliance with regulatory requirements.
4. **Professional Reputation:** High-quality practices enhance the reputation of healthcare facilities and professionals.

Conclusion:

Quality assurance and error prevention are integral to laboratory testing, safeguarding patient safety, and ensuring accurate results. Phlebotomists' commitment to standardized procedures, meticulous attention to detail, and vigilant error prevention strategies uphold the integrity of the testing process. By adhering to these principles, phlebotomists contribute to the overall quality of healthcare delivery, patient outcomes, and the credibility of laboratory practices.

Phlebotomy, the art and science of blood collection, is a critical step in laboratory testing. The accuracy and reliability of diagnostic results hinge on the quality of phlebotomy procedures and the meticulous attention to detail exhibited by phlebotomists. Ensuring quality in phlebotomy procedures is essential to maintaining patient safety, preventing errors, and upholding laboratory practice standards.

In this section, we look into the fundamental principles and practices that underpin quality in phlebotomy procedures. From patient interaction to specimen collection, handling, and transportation, every aspect of the phlebotomy process plays a role in the accuracy of laboratory testing outcomes. By emphasizing adherence to protocols, patient-centered care, and error prevention strategies, this section empowers phlebotomists to consistently deliver high-quality results and contribute to the overall excellence of healthcare services.

1. Preventing Pre-Analytical Errors

Pre-analytical errors, which occur before the actual laboratory analysis, can significantly impact the accuracy and reliability of test results. These errors can stem from various stages of the phlebotomy process, from patient identification to specimen collection and handling. In this section, we explore the crucial strategies and best

practices for preventing pre-analytical errors in phlebotomy,
emphasizing the importance of patient safety, specimen integrity,
and meticulous attention to detail.

Pre-analytical errors encompass a wide range of potential mistakes,
including misidentification of patients, improper specimen labeling,
contamination, and mishandling. These errors can lead to incorrect
diagnoses, inappropriate treatments, and compromised patient care.
By focusing on error prevention at every stage of the pre-analytical
process, phlebotomists contribute to accurate and reliable laboratory
testing outcomes.

Strategies for Preventing Pre-Analytical Errors:
1. **Patient Identification:** Verify patient identity using at least
   two unique identifiers (e.g., name, date of birth) before
   collecting blood.
2. **Specimen Labeling:** Ensure accurate and legible labeling of
   specimens immediately after collection, using the patient's
   information.
3. **Patient Preparation:** Instruct patients on necessary
   preparations, such as fasting or medication restrictions, to
   avoid sample interference.
4. **Proper Phlebotomy Techniques:** Adhere to established
   venipuncture techniques to minimize discomfort, risk of
   contamination, and complications.
5. **Specimen Integrity:** Use appropriate collection tubes and

ensure proper anticoagulant-to-blood ratio to maintain specimen integrity.

6. **Minimizing Hemolysis:** Handle specimens gently and avoid excessive agitation to prevent hemolysis, which can impact test results.

7. **Contamination Prevention:** Follow aseptic techniques to prevent contamination of specimens, collection equipment, and work areas.

8. **Proper Transport and Storage:** Use appropriate containers for transporting and storing specimens, maintaining temperature stability.

9. **Documentation Accuracy:** Accurately document patient information, collection times, and any deviations from standard procedures.

Benefits of Preventing Pre-Analytical Errors:

1. **Patient Safety:** Error prevention safeguards patient safety by ensuring accurate diagnoses and appropriate treatments.

2. **Reliable Results:** Quality pre-analytical practices contribute to the reliability and credibility of laboratory test results.

3. **Effective Healthcare:** Accurate results guide healthcare decisions, enhancing the effectiveness of patient care and interventions.

4. **Cost Efficiency:** Reducing errors minimizes the need for retesting, conserving resources, and reducing healthcare costs.

Conclusion:

Preventing pre-analytical errors is an integral part of phlebotomy practice that directly impacts patient safety and the quality of laboratory testing outcomes. By diligently adhering to protocols, employing error prevention strategies, and prioritizing patient-centered care, phlebotomists play a pivotal role in ensuring specimens' accuracy, reliability, and integrity. Embracing these practices reflects a commitment to excellence, patient well-being, and the foundational principles of quality in phlebotomy.

2. Documentation and Record Keeping

Accurate and comprehensive documentation is a cornerstone of phlebotomy practice that ensures proper patient care, traceability, and the integrity of laboratory testing processes. Thorough record-keeping supports error prevention and facilitates effective communication among healthcare team members. In this section, we delve into the significance of documentation and record-keeping in phlebotomy, the essential elements to include, and their role in maintaining patient safety and the quality of healthcare services.

Documentation is a vital link in the continuum of patient care and laboratory testing. Accurate records provide a chronological account of the phlebotomy process, from patient identification and preparation to specimen collection, handling, and transport. These records enable healthcare professionals to track patient progress and maintain accountability for every step of the procedure.

Essential Elements of Documentation:

1. **Patient Identification:** Document the patient's full name, date of birth, and unique identifiers to prevent errors.

2. **Collection Date and Time:** Record the exact date and time of specimen collection to ensure accuracy and traceability.

3. **Test Requisition:** Include information about the tests requested by the physician, ensuring that the appropriate tests are performed.

4. **Specimen Details:** Document the type of specimen collected, the site of collection, and the volume collected.

5. **Phlebotomist Identification:** Identify the phlebotomist responsible for the collection, ensuring accountability.

6. **Patient Preparation:** Note any patient-specific preparations, such as fasting or medication restrictions.

7. **Special Considerations:** Document any challenges or deviations encountered during the phlebotomy process.

8. **Patient Consent:** Record patient consent for specific procedures or tests if applicable.

Role of Documentation in Patient Safety:

1. **Error Prevention:** Accurate documentation helps prevent errors by providing clear instructions for each step of the phlebotomy process.

2. **Patient Identification:** Proper documentation ensures that patients are correctly identified, reducing the risk of misidentification.

3. **Communication:** Clear records facilitate effective communication among healthcare team members, ensuring coordinated care.

4. **Treatment Decision-Making:** Accurate documentation guides healthcare providers in making informed treatment decisions based on reliable data.

Benefits of Effective Record Keeping:

1. **Patient-Centered Care:** Comprehensive records support patient-centered care by ensuring continuity and accuracy in treatment.

2. **Legal and Regulatory Compliance:** Thorough documentation fulfills legal and regulatory requirements, ensuring accountability.

3. **Data Integrity:** Accurate records contribute to the integrity of laboratory testing data and ensure its reliability.

4. **Quality Assurance:** Proper documentation supports quality assurance efforts, demonstrating adherence to best practices.

Conclusion:

Documentation and record keeping are integral aspects of phlebotomy practice that uphold patient safety, accountability, and the quality of healthcare services. By accurately documenting every aspect of the phlebotomy process, from patient identification to specimen handling, phlebotomists contribute to error prevention, effective communication, and overall patient care excellence.

Embracing meticulous documentation practices reflects a commitment to professionalism, patient well-being, and the highest standards of phlebotomy practice.

Professionalism and Ethical Behavior

Professionalism and ethical behavior are fundamental attributes for phlebotomists that define their interactions with patients, colleagues, and the healthcare system. These qualities encompass a commitment to integrity, respect, patient confidentiality, and the highest standards of practice. In this section, we explore the significance of professionalism and ethical behavior in phlebotomy, their impact on patient care and trust, and their role in upholding the integrity of the healthcare profession.

Professionalism goes beyond technical skills; it embodies the values, attitudes, and behaviors that reflect a phlebotomist's dedication to patient-centered care and ethical principles. Ethical behavior ensures that patients' rights are respected, their information is kept confidential, and their well-being is prioritized. These qualities build trust between patients and healthcare providers and contribute to a positive healthcare experience.

Key Aspects of Professionalism and Ethical Behavior:
1. **Patient-Centered Care:** Prioritize patients' needs, comfort, and safety throughout phlebotomy.
2. **Respect and Empathy:** Treat patients, colleagues, and healthcare team members with respect and empathy.
3. **Integrity:** Uphold honesty and transparency in all interactions, ensuring accuracy and truthfulness in

communication.

4. **Confidentiality:** Safeguard patient confidentiality by adhering to strict confidentiality protocols.

5. **Continuous Learning:** Engage in ongoing education and professional development to stay updated on best practices.

6. **Accountability:** Take responsibility for actions and decisions, striving for excellence in all aspects of practice.

7. **Adherence to Standards:** Follow established guidelines, protocols, and regulations to ensure patient safety.

Impact on Patient Care and Trust:

1. **Patient Trust:** Professionalism and ethical behavior foster trust between patients and phlebotomists, enhancing the patient-provider relationship.

2. **Positive Experience:** Patient-centered care and respectful interactions create a positive healthcare experience.

3. **Confidentiality:** Ethical handling of patient information fosters confidence in the security of personal data.

4. **Effective Communication:** Clear, respectful communication builds understanding and encourages patient cooperation.

Benefits of Professionalism and Ethical Behavior:

1. **Patient Safety:** Ethical behavior and professionalism contribute to accurate and safe patient care.

2. **Healthcare Reputation:** Upholding high ethical standards enhances the reputation of healthcare facilities and

professionals.

3. **Personal Fulfillment:** Demonstrating professionalism brings personal satisfaction and pride in delivering high-quality care.

Conclusion:

Professionalism and ethical behavior form the foundation of phlebotomy practice, shaping how phlebotomists interact with patients, colleagues, and the healthcare system. By embodying these attributes, phlebotomists create a supportive and trustworthy environment for patients and contribute to the integrity and credibility of the healthcare profession. Striving for professionalism and ethical conduct upholds healthcare values and ensures patients receive the highest standard of care and respect they deserve.

1. Continuing Education and Certifications

Continuing education and certifications are indispensable components of a phlebotomist's professional journey, enabling them to stay current with evolving healthcare practices and maintain the highest standards of competence. In this section, we explore the vital role of continuing education, the significance of certifications, and how these efforts contribute to the growth of phlebotomists' knowledge, skills, and overall effectiveness in patient care.

New techniques, technologies, and best practices continually emerge in the dynamic healthcare field. Continuing education ensures that phlebotomists remain well-informed about the latest advancements and changes, allowing them to provide the best possible care to their patients. By staying updated, phlebotomists enhance their clinical competence, adapt to evolving protocols, and contribute to improving healthcare services.

Benefits of Continuing Education:

1. **Clinical Excellence:** Continuing education equips phlebotomists with the latest knowledge and techniques, enhancing their clinical skills and expertise.
2. **Patient Safety:** Staying current with best practices ensures patients receive the safest and most effective care.
3. **Adaptability:** Continuous learning prepares phlebotomists to adapt to changes in healthcare practices, technologies, and regulations.
4. **Career Advancement:** Updated skills and knowledge can open doors to new opportunities and career advancement.

The Significance of Certifications:

Certifications validate a phlebotomist's competence and expertise in the field, providing a recognized standard of proficiency. Becoming certified demonstrates a commitment to professionalism and excellence in practice, enhancing one's credibility as a healthcare professional. Various certification programs, such as those offered by professional organizations, validate a phlebotomist's knowledge, skills, and adherence to ethical standards.

Benefits of Certifications:

1. **Credibility:** Certifications demonstrate that phlebotomists have met established standards of practice and possess a high level of competence.

2. **Employment Opportunities:** Many healthcare employers require or prefer certified phlebotomists, expanding job prospects.

3. **Professional Growth:** Certifications can lead to increased responsibilities, recognition, and advancement in the healthcare field.

4. **Patient Trust:** Certification instills patient trust, assuring they receive care from a qualified and certified professional.

Embracing a Lifelong Learning Mindset:

Continuing education and certifications are not one-time achievements but ongoing commitments to lifelong learning. Embracing this mindset allows phlebotomists to continually refine their skills, expand their knowledge, and adapt to the ever-evolving healthcare landscape.

Conclusion:

Continuing education and certifications are integral to the professional journey of a phlebotomist. By staying informed, honing their skills, and earning certifications, phlebotomists not only enhance their professional growth but also contribute to improving patient care, the credibility of their profession, and the overall advancement of healthcare practices. A commitment to continuous learning reflects a dedication to excellence and a passion for providing the highest quality care to patients.

2. Job Opportunities and Career Advancement

Phlebotomy offers a dynamic and rewarding career path with diverse job opportunities and avenues for advancement within the healthcare field. A skilled phlebotomist is vital in patient care, diagnostic processes, and laboratory operations. In this section, we explore the range of job opportunities available to phlebotomists, the potential for career advancement, and the factors contributing to a successful and fulfilling professional journey.

Phlebotomists are in demand across various healthcare settings, including hospitals, clinics, laboratories, blood banks, and diagnostic centers. Their role extends beyond blood collection to specimen handling, patient interaction, and collaboration with healthcare teams. Phlebotomists may also specialize in specific areas, such as pediatric or geriatric phlebotomy, enhancing their skills and qualifications.

Career Pathways and Advancement:

Phlebotomy serves as a stepping stone to numerous career pathways within healthcare. As phlebotomists gain experience and expand their skill set, opportunities for career advancement become available. Some possible pathways include:

1. **Lead Phlebotomist:** Lead phlebotomists supervise and coordinate the work of other phlebotomists, ensuring smooth operations and quality control.

2. **Laboratory Technician:** With additional training, phlebotomists can become laboratory technicians, performing a more comprehensive range of laboratory tasks.

3. **Medical Laboratory Scientist/Technologist:** Further education and certification can lead to roles as medical laboratory scientists or technologists, with responsibilities spanning various laboratory procedures and analyses.

4. **Healthcare Administration:** With experience, phlebotomists can transition into administrative roles, such as healthcare supervisors or managers.

Factors Contributing to Career Success:

1. **Skill Development:** Continuously honing technical skills and expanding knowledge enhances career growth.

2. **Certifications:** Earning certifications showcases expertise and opens doors to more advanced roles.

3. **Communication Skills:** Effective communication with patients, colleagues, and healthcare teams enhances job performance.

4. **Adaptability:** Adapting to new technologies and evolving healthcare practices is crucial for long-term success.

5. **Ethical Behavior:** Demonstrating professionalism and ethical behavior fosters trust and career advancement.

6. **Networking:** Building professional relationships within the healthcare community can create new opportunities.

Personal Fulfillment and Job Satisfaction:

A career in phlebotomy is not only financially rewarding but also personally fulfilling. The direct impact on patient care, the opportunity to work in a dynamic healthcare environment, and the potential for career advancement contribute to job satisfaction and a sense of purpose.

Conclusion:

Phlebotomy offers a fulfilling and diverse career path with ample job opportunities and the potential for growth within the healthcare industry. Phlebotomists can carve out a successful and fulfilling career journey by continuously improving skills, seeking certifications, and embracing new challenges. As integral healthcare team members, phlebotomists contribute to patient well-being, the accuracy of medical diagnoses, and the overall excellence of healthcare services.

Appendices

A. Glossary of Phlebotomy Terms

This glossary provides definitions and explanations for essential terms and phrases used in phlebotomy. It is a comprehensive reference to help readers understand the specialized terminology associated with blood collection, specimen handling, laboratory testing, and related practices.

1. **Anticoagulant:** A substance added to blood collection tubes to prevent clotting and maintain the integrity of blood samples.

2. **Capillary Puncture:** The process of collecting blood from a small prick in the skin, typically using a lancet, for specific tests or in cases where venipuncture is challenging.

3. **Hematoma:** A localized swelling filled with blood that occurs when blood leaks into surrounding tissues during or after venipuncture.

4. **Informed Consent:** The process of obtaining permission from a patient before performing a medical procedure, ensuring that they understand the procedure, its risks, and benefits.

5. **Phlebotomist:** A healthcare professional trained in blood collection techniques, responsible for obtaining blood specimens from patients for laboratory testing.

6. **Specimen:** A sample of blood, urine, tissue, or other bodily fluids collected for laboratory analysis and diagnosis.

7. **Tourniquet:** A device temporarily constricts blood flow in a vein, making veins more visible and accessible during venipuncture.

8. **Venipuncture:** The process of puncturing a vein with a needle to collect blood for diagnostic testing or medical treatment.

9. **Hemolysis:** The breakdown or destruction of red blood cells, often resulting from rough handling of blood specimens or improper collection techniques.

10. **Needle Gauge:** A measurement indicating the diameter of a needle; smaller gauge numbers represent larger needles.

11. **Hematology:** The branch of medical science deals with blood study, including its formation, composition, and diseases.

12. **Serum:** The clear liquid portion of blood obtained after coagulation, often used for various diagnostic tests.

13. **Plasma:** The liquid component of blood that remains when blood cells are removed, containing water, electrolytes, and proteins.

14. **Infection Control:** Practices and protocols aimed at preventing the spread of infections within healthcare settings, including proper hand hygiene and personal protective equipment usage.

15. **Patient Identification Band:** A wristband or identification tag used to ensure accurate patient identification during the collection of blood specimens.

This glossary is valuable for students studying for a phlebotomy exam and professionals seeking to enhance their understanding of key terms and concepts in the field.

B. Common Abbreviations in Phlebotomy

The following list presents commonly used abbreviations in phlebotomy, aiding readers in quickly interpreting medical documents, charts, and communication-related to blood collection and laboratory testing.

1. **CBC**: Complete Blood Count
2. **PT**: Prothrombin Time
3. **PTT**: Partial Thromboplastin Time
4. **INR**: International Normalized Ratio
5. **HbA1c**: Hemoglobin A1c
6. **RBC**: Red Blood Cell Count
7. **WBC**: White Blood Cell Count
8. **Hct**: Hematocrit
9. **PLT**: Platelet Count
10. **UA**: Urinalysis
11. **BUN**: Blood Urea Nitrogen
12. **ESR**: Erythrocyte Sedimentation Rate
13. **CMP**: Comprehensive Metabolic Panel
14. **HIV**: Human Immunodeficiency Virus
15. **HBV**: Hepatitis B Virus
16. **HCV**: Hepatitis C Virus

17. **PPE**: Personal Protective Equipment

18. **CDC**: Centers for Disease Control and Prevention

19. **HIPAA**: Health Insurance Portability and Accountability Act

20. **CLIA**: Clinical Laboratory Improvement Amendments

21. **OSHA**: Occupational Safety and Health Administration

These abbreviations are convenient tools for communication, documentation, and interpretation within phlebotomy and laboratory testing. Familiarity with these abbreviations enhances efficiency and accuracy in the healthcare environment.

Tales of Phlebotomy

Case #1: The Order of Death

The morning began like any other for Richard and Margaret, who were finally retired and ready to finish living their life together. Richard had worked for the same company for over 40 years. He had just gotten out of bed to shower while his wife Margaret started his morning coffee. Richard was getting ready for his monthly check-up with his doctor.

"Lover! Are you almost finished? Your coffee is getting cold!" Margaret shouted from the kitchen.

Richard entered the kitchen and sat at the breakfast table with his coffee and paper before his doctor's appointment.

Richard reached over and gently grabbed his wife's hand and said, "So, my love, what do you want to do this weekend?"

"I don't know. Maybe we should finally visit the grandkids. We haven't seen them in almost a year." Margaret replied.

"Okay, that sounds like a good idea. Let me get to my doctor's appointment and make sure this new medication is working. Then we can plan the trip for this weekend."

Richard finished his coffee and headed to his appointment. On the way, Richard stopped by the donut shop to pick up a few dozen donuts for the staff as he did every appointment.

He pulled up to his doctor's office, just a few miles from his home, and parked in the same handicap spot for years. Richard grabbed his cane and donuts and headed over to the medical building. He walked in, and a few nurses and staff called out, "Hi Richard! How are you doing this morning? It's good to see you again."

Richard looked at them with a big smile and said, "I am doing great this morning, thank you. It is wonderful to see you all this morning, too."

Richard walked over to the sign-in sheet and handed the donuts to the young girl behind the counter.

"Thank you, Richard; you never forget, do you?" The young girl said.

"You are very welcome; it is my pleasure," Richard replied. Richard walked over to the waiting area and sat down to wait for his doctor.

After about 45 minutes, the nurse opened the door and called Richard back to see the doctor. Richard walked back with the nurse to the exam room and sat down on the exam table to wait for the doctor to come. The nurse saw his nervousness and said, "So, what are you and your wife doing this weekend?" Hoping to make him less nervous.

"Well, the wife and I are going to plan a trip to visit our grandkids who live out of state," Richard replied. "We haven't seen them in almost a year, and we miss them very much."

"Oh, how wonderful!" The nurse responded. "Well, you sit there, and the doctor will be in shortly to see you." She said as she slowly closed the door behind her.

After about another 30 minutes, the doctor walked in and said, "Good morning Richard, how are you doing this morning? How are the kids and grandkids?"

"Oh, they are doing great. The wife and I are planning to visit them this weekend. It has been almost a year since we have seen them." Richard repeated.

"Wonderful!" The doctor responded. "Well, let's see if the new medication I prescribed for your heart is working. I will have someone draw your blood to see if everything is normal."

"Sounds great, doc!" Richard replied.

While he was waiting to get his blood drawn, he was thinking about his trip with his wife. The places they were going to stop and visit along the way, and the surprise he was planning for his wife on the trip. He was working out all the details for their journey together.

At that moment, the phlebotomist walked in to draw his blood. "Hello, the doctor ordered some blood work. Is it okay if I draw your blood?" The phlebotomist asked.

"Yes, of course," Richard responded.

"Okay, great. Can you please tell me your first and last name with spelling?" She asked.

Richard began to give her all the information she requested to draw his blood.

The phlebotomist drew his blood and sent it to the lab for the results. At that moment, the doctor walked into the exam room and said, "Okay, Richard, it should take about an hour to get the results. Go ahead and take a seat in the waiting room, and I will call you back when the results are finished."

"Okay, doc. Thank you." Richard responded as he made his way back to the waiting room.

After about an hour, the nurse opened the door and called Richard back to the exam room to see the doctor for the blood test results.

"Okay, Richard, this is what I see from the results." The doctor started to say. "It looks like your potassium level is higher than I want for you. So, I will lower the dose of your medication to help bring it down to a normal level." The doctor explained.

"Okay, doc, whatever you say. I want to be healthy for my weekend trip with my wife." Richard responded.

The doctor gave him another prescription to get filled at the drugstore on the way home.

When Richard arrived home with his new medication, his wife had lunch ready for him to eat. "Hello, love," Richard said to his wife.

"Well, how did it go?" His wife responded and asked.

"The doctor ran some blood tests and said my potassium is high, so he gave me some new medication to help make it normal again," Richard told his wife as he sat down to eat lunch.

"Oh, good. As long as you are better for this weekend. I can't wait to go up and visit the kids." She said to her husband. "Now eat your lunch and take the pills the doctor gave you."

Richard finished his lunch and got up to kiss his wife on the cheek. "I am going to take my pills and nap." He told his wife.

"Okay, but don't sleep too long. We need to pack and plan the drive for this weekend." She told Richard.

Richard was excited because he had already planned a few surprises for Margaret along the way on the drive.

"I won't. I'll set the alarm to wake me up." He told his wife.

Margaret decided to go outside and work in the garden while her husband napped. After a few hours, she noticed that Richard had not awakened yet. As she started to head back to the house from the garden, she stopped and cleaned herself up from the dirt on her hands and shoes. She rinsed her hands and shoes from the water hose outside.

As she entered the house, she shouted, "Richard, honey, are you awake!" There was no response.

She started walking to the bedroom, where Richard was napping. She opened the bedroom door and said, "Richard, love, it is time to wake up. It's getting late." There was still no response.

She walked toward the side of the bed where he was sleeping, touched his arm, and said, "Richard? Wake up, dear. We need to get ready for the trip this weekend." There was still no response from Richard.

At that moment, she began to panic and shout, "Richard, wake up! What is wrong?" As she began to shake him to wake up.

Richard was not responding to her. At that moment, she ran to the phone in the kitchen to call 911. She told the 911 operator that her husband was not waking up. The operator sent the paramedics to their house immediately.

The ambulance rushed Richard to the hospital while his wife followed behind in her car. When she arrived at the hospital, Richard was still not responding.

After about an hour, the doctor came out to the waiting room where Margaret was sitting and waiting for any news about her husband.

The doctor approached Margaret, put his head down, and said, "I am sorry, Margaret. Richard did not make it."

At that moment, her eyes began to water. "What do you mean he did not make it? He was fine this morning before he came to see you." She said while trying to hold back her tears.

"I am truly sorry, Margaret." The doctor replied.

At that moment, Margaret realized her greatest fear. She had lost her husband and partner for life. She never imagined the love of her life would die so early. They both were only 62 years old. She would now have to tell their kids and grandkids that their dad and grandpa had died. But why? What happened? How could Richard die so suddenly after his routine doctor visit?

WHAT HAPPENED?

Before his blood draw, let's examine what happened to Richard at the doctor's office. When the doctor saw Richard in the exam room and told him he would order some blood work, a new phlebotomist was on duty. This phlebotomist had just graduated two months earlier and only worked for about a week at the office.

When the doctor left the exam room, he told the phlebotomist to draw blood for a complete blood count, known as a CBC, and potassium levels in exam room 3. This would require a lavender top tube containing the additive EDTA and a green top tube containing heparin.

When the phlebotomist was preparing her stuff to draw Richard in exam room 3, she asked the nurse if it mattered in what order she drew the tubes while getting the blood.

"No, it doesn't matter. Just get the blood." The nurse responded.

This response leads to a chain of events that ultimately cost Richard his life. The EDTA tube that the phlebotomist used is high in potassium by nature. So, when she used the EDTA tube first instead of the green heparin tube, as required by the *Order of Draw* in phlebotomy, the additive carried over into the green tube when she used it after the lavender tube. This caused the potassium to seem elevated when Richard had normal potassium levels already because of the current medication he was taking.

When the doctor received the test results, he noticed the spike in Richard's potassium due to the phlebotomist not following the correct draw order. The doctor then decides to lower Richard's medication even though it is unnecessary. Richard gets his new medication, which lowers his already normal potassium level. This is called hypokalemia.

Potassium is an electrolyte, and it transmits electrical impulses through the heart as well as to other muscles. Hypokalemia can disrupt nerve impulses that travel through the heart and cause it to contract. This decrease in potassium can cause poor contraction when it is low in the body. If this happens, the person can go into cardiac arrest, which was the case with Richard after he took the new medication right before his nap.

If the nurse and the phlebotomist had been appropriately trained about the order of draw, Richard would still be alive today, visiting his family with his wife. This tragedy did not have to happen to Richard and his family. Instead, he received the order of death.

Case #2: To Tear or NOT to Tear?

Doug and Lisa were expecting their first child. They have been trying to conceive for almost three years. During that time, Lisa had two miscarriages. It has been a long and challenging road for both of them. Doug and Lisa are getting everything ready with only one month to go.

"Doug! Did you remember to get the baby's diapers and wipes at the store?" Lisa asked.

"Yes, dear. I got everything on the list you gave me." Doug responded.

"I am just so excited. Our little baby girl will be here with us in one month." Lisa said while starting to tear up.

"I know. We have been trying for so long, and our prayers have been answered. We are so blessed." Doug responded as he kissed and hugged Lisa.

"I am just so emotional right now. I didn't think I could get pregnant after we lost the first two." Lisa said as she was starting to cry.

A few days later, both their parents came by their house to visit and bring extra baby supplies.

"Oh, we are so excited to meet our new granddaughter!" Doug's parents said with joy.

"Oh yes, I can't wait to hold and love her every day." Lisa's parents replied. This would be the first grandchild for both parents.

Doug and Lisa were getting everything ready in the baby's room for the next two weeks. Their daughter's arrival was getting closer and closer.

One morning, Lisa woke up, turned to Doug, and said, "Honey, wake up. I think it's time."

"Are you sure?" Doug asked.

"Yes, my water just broke," Lisa responded with nervousness.

Doug jumped out of bed, grabbed their overnight bag, and helped Lisa to the car. He drove quickly to the hospital, which was about 20 minutes away. Both were nervous and excited at the same time.

When they arrived at the hospital, Doug helped Lisa into the wheelchair while the nurse asked how far along she was in the pregnancy.

"I'm 36 weeks, and my water just broke," Lisa answered.

"Okay, let's get you into a room so the doctor can examine you." The nurse replied.

The nurse took Lisa to the hospital's Labor and Delivery area and started taking her vitals before the doctor arrived.

"Everything looks good." The nurse said to Lisa and Doug.

A few minutes late, the doctor came into the room. "Good morning, you two. How are you feeling, Lisa?" The doctor asked.

"I am feeling okay. I'm feeling a lot of contractions happening in a short time." Lisa responded.

The doctor checked Lisa and the baby to make sure everything was okay.

"Well, everything looks good. You and the baby are doing great. You are dilated to 7." The doctor told Lisa.

Within a few hours, Lisa gave birth to a 6.5-pound baby girl named Emma. The whole family came to the hospital to see Lisa and Emma.

"Congratulations!" Everyone would say when they saw Lisa and Doug with Emma.

Doug and Lisa took baby Emma to her new home within a couple of days. Both grandparents were there waiting to hold and love baby Emma. The next few weeks were the happiest days for Doug and Lisa.

One day, Lisa noticed that Emma had a little cold. So, she went to the kitchen to get some cold medicine for Emma. The next day, Emma woke up with a fever of 102. Lisa started to get worried, so she called Doug at work.

"Honey, Emma has a fever of 102, and I gave her medicine, but it hasn't gone down," Lisa told Doug.

"Okay, go ahead and take her to see the doctor at the hospital," Doug said.

Lisa drove baby Emma to the hospital where she was born to see their doctor.

Lisa checked baby Emma into the hospital and told the nurse what had happened. The nurse took baby Emma's vitals and confirmed that she still had a fever. The nurse put baby Emma and Lisa into an examining room and told Lisa to wait until the doctor could come in to see Emma.

When the doctor entered the examiner's room, he said, "Hello, you two. What seems to be wrong?" As he started to examine baby Emma.

"Well, Emma woke up this morning with a little cold but got a fever too. I gave her some cold medicine, but the fever would not go down. I worried, and Doug told me to bring her to see you." Lisa explained to the doctor.

"Okay. She still has a high fever. I will order some blood tests and admit her until we can see the results. Then we can see what is wrong." The doctor told Lisa.

The doctor admitted baby Emma while Lisa called Doug to tell him what happened.

"It will be okay, honey. Emma is in good hands. The doctor will take good care of her." Doug told Lisa.

"I know, but I am just worried about Emma," Lisa told Doug.

After a few hours, the doctor saw Lisa and Emma. "Okay, the blood tests show that Emma has a viral infection causing the cold and fever." The doctor explained to Lisa. "We will keep her for a few more hours and get the fever down with medication. After that, she will be fine to take home." The doctor said.

"Oh, thank goodness!" Lisa told the doctor with happiness in her voice. "I will call Doug and tell him the good news," Lisa told the doctor.

Lisa went outside to call Doug and let him know what was happening with Emma. "Oh, thank God!" Doug told Lisa. "I was starting to get a little worried, too," Doug explained to Lisa.

"I know. One minute, she is happy and playing at home; the next, she is at the hospital." Lisa told Doug.

"It will be okay, honey. The doctor said she would be fine in a few hours. Then you can retake her home." Doug responded.

After a few hours, the doctor came into the room to speak to Lisa with a concerned look.

"What is wrong, doctor?" Lisa asked.

"Emma is not responding to the medication we gave her. We continued to give her antibiotics, but they are not working." The doctor explained to Lisa.

"What do you mean the antibiotics are not working? Why would it not work?" Lisa asked.

"The infection is spreading to her lungs and seems resistant to our strongest antibiotics." The doctor explained to Lisa.

"How could this happen? What could cause this infection?" Lisa asked while starting to worry.

"We are not sure yet. We still are running more tests. We are doing everything we can for Emma. I am sorry." The doctor told Lisa with a sad voice.

Lisa immediately called Doug and told him what was happening to Emma. Doug left work and rushed to the hospital to be with Lisa while the doctor moved baby Emma to the ICU. Within a few hours, baby Emma died from a bacterial infection called CRE that she acquired while at the hospital. After three years of trying to have their first child, Doug and Lisa's greatest fear happened. Nothing could prepare them for the loss of baby Emma.

WHAT HAPPENED?

Let us examine what happened before the doctor ordered blood work on baby Emma when she was hospitalized for a cold and fever. What should have been a simple blood draw from the phlebotomist turned into a parent's worst nightmare.

The lab in the hospital was backed up that afternoon with blood draw orders. There was only one phlebotomist on duty at the time. Two other phlebotomists called off work just before their shift started. There was no time to get coverage until later in the evening.

The phlebotomist on duty that day was running from department to department to finish her blood draws on patients waiting for hours. She was a 20-year veteran in the field of phlebotomy. She was trained in the old ways of doing blood draws.

After the doctor examined Emma, he called the lab and sent them orders to draw baby Emma's blood for tests. The phlebotomist, who was alone that evening, received the order after drawing a dozen patients just earlier. She quickly went to the examiner's room to draw baby Emma. When she entered the room, Lisa stepped out to call Doug about Emma's condition while the doctor was getting Emma admitted.

The phlebotomist failed to wash her hands before handling baby Emma. She put on her gloves and gathered equipment to draw Emma's blood from her arm. The phlebotomist was having difficulty feeling Emma's vein on her arm. So, the phlebotomist decided to tear off a piece of the glove on her finger so she could feel the vein better on Emma's arm. Emma was sick, and her immune system was weak and underdeveloped as a newborn.

The unwashed and exposed finger of the phlebotomist touching baby Emma's arm just before she stuck her with a needle caused Emma to be exposed to a super antibiotic-resistant bacterium called CRE.

When a patient is exposed to CRE in the blood, it is almost impossible to treat effectively.

Nobody saw that the phlebotomist did not wash her hands before putting on her gloves or that she tore off a piece of the glove from her finger just before touching Emma's arm. The phlebotomist was not trained and updated on the current standard of care set by the governing phlebotomy agencies.

This tragedy could have been easily avoided if the phlebotomist had taken the time to wash her hands before entering the room or if she had not touched a patient without personal protective equipment. In this case, "not" tearing off a piece of her glove from her finger. Those simple actions could have saved baby Emma's life.

Doug and Lisa's life will never be the same after losing their first and maybe their only child. Nobody should have to bury their newborn child because of a phlebotomist's senseless and careless action. They will not be able to see their child grow up and live the life she was supposed to.

Case #3: The Three "Ps"

Samantha is a 23-year-old college student who just made the track team. This would include a full scholarship and tryouts at the next Olympics. She has been dreaming of this opportunity for her whole life. She grew up in a small town and is the youngest of 4 children.

One morning, Samantha woke up with bad stomach cramps. She was holding her stomach, groaning in pain.

"Are you okay?" Samantha's roommate Sarah asked.

"I don't know. My stomach is killing me." Samantha replied.

"Maybe it was all that junk food you ate last night," Sarah said while grinning.

"Maybe. Do you have any stomach pain medicine I can take?" Samantha asked Sarah.

"Let me check," Sarah replied.

Sarah went into the bathroom to look for medicine to help Samantha.

"Here, try this antacid and see if it helps," Sarah said while handing Samantha the medicine.

Samantha took the antacid medicine and went back to bed to rest for about an hour.

After a couple of hours, Sarah checked on Samantha in her bedroom.

"How are you feeling, Sam?" Sarah asked.

"My stomach is still killing me," Samantha replied.

"Then we need to take you to the emergency room and make sure you are okay. Something could be very wrong with you, Sam," Sarah told her.

"Okay. This pain is just too much to deal with right now." Samantha replied.

Sarah helped Samantha out of bed and walked her down to the car outside. The hospital was only a few miles away. Samantha was curled up in the backseat of the car in pain.

"Hang on, Sam. We will be there soon." Sarah told her.

When Samantha got to the hospital, the nurse gave her some pain medication that helped her stomach until the doctor saw her in the exam room.

"Hello, Samantha; what seems to be the problem?" The doctor asked as he walked into the room.

"I woke up this morning with bad stomach pain. I tried taking an antacid, but it didn't work." She replied.

"Okay. I will order some blood work, and then we will take an ultrasound of your stomach and see what is happening there." The doctor responded as he left the room.

About an hour later, the phlebotomist came into the room to draw her blood while she was sitting up on the exam table. The phlebotomist drew her blood and left the room to return it to the lab.

About another hour passed before the doctor returned to the exam, where he found Samantha bleeding from her head on the floor. The doctor immediately called the nurses to help get Samantha up and into a bed. Samantha had fractured her head along with several vertebrae.

The x-ray and tests confirmed that she was now paralyzed and could no longer walk. She would use a wheelchair for the rest of her life. Samantha's dream of competing in the Olympics was now over—another tragedy from a simple blood draw.

WHAT HAPPENED?

Let us examine what happened after the doctor ordered some blood tests for Samantha. When the phlebotomist came in the room an hour after the doctor left, Samantha was sitting on the edge of the exam table. The phlebotomist introduced herself and asked Samantha to say her full name with spelling.

After the phlebotomist checked the information with the requisition, she began to draw Samantha's blood from her arm while she was sitting up on the exam table. The phlebotomist quickly left the room after she had finished, and Samantha slowly passed out within a minute while sitting on the table's edge. She fell off the exam table headfirst onto the floor, where she fractured her skull and vertebrae.

The phlebotomist failed to make sure that Samantha was okay after the blood draw. If the phlebotomist had asked Samantha the three "Ps," she would have known that Samantha has a history of feeling faint after a blood draw.

So, what are the three "Ps" the phlebotomist should have asked Samantha?

1. **Patient's ID**-first and last name is spelled out by the patient.
2. **Patient complication**-light headed or fainting in the past.
3. **Patient medication**-blood-thinners

The phlebotomist asked for the patient's ID. However, she did not ask Samantha if she ever had any complications while having her blood drawn. That question would have let the phlebotomist know that Samantha gets light-headed during a blood draw. The phlebotomist would have laid her down on the exam table while she drew her blood. This would have saved Samantha from falling headfirst onto the floor and getting paralyzed by the injury after the blood draw.

The last "P" is for patients on certain blood thinners. The phlebotomist must know if the patient might bleed out after the blood draw. The pressure applied after will have to be longer on the draw site than the average time. This can prevent the patient from losing too much blood and passing out while standing.

The simple three "P" questions could literally save a patient's life. In this case, Samantha was not so lucky. She will spend the rest of her life in a wheelchair, and her dreams are no longer a reality but only dreams again.

Case #4: What "Nerve"

Sally was a successful dentist who looked forward to seeing her patients every day at her office. Her patients loved her because she took good care of them. Sally was recognized in her city as one of the top dentists in the state. It would be a routine yearly physical that would be her worst nightmare.

Sally started her day like any other day on the morning of her physical. She took her morning shower and headed downstairs for breakfast with her husband, Steve, and her two kids, Noah and Sarah.

"Good morning, dear. Do you have another busy day with patients?" Her husband asked.

"I don't have too many today. I have my yearly physical later today." She responded.

"Oh, good. So, you should be home early for dinner with the kids and me?" Steve asked.

"It does look like I should have a simple day and be home for dinner early." She responded.

"Great! If anything changes, give me a call." Steve said.

After breakfast, Sally kissed her husband and kids goodbye and headed to her office.

As Sally arrived at her office, one of her regular patients was waiting outside for her office with a box of muffins for her and her staff.

As Sally exited her car, she said, "Hi, Freddy! How are you doing today?"

"I am great, Sally! I feel wonderful today." Freddy responded.

Freddy was an 86-year-old man who only trusted Sally to work on his teeth. Many of Sally's patients only came to her for dental work.

At about noon, Sally started to get ready to go to her yearly physical with her doctor. She left her office and drove about 35 minutes away to see her doctor. As Sally arrived and entered her doctor's office, she was greeted by the front desk medical assistant.

"Good afternoon Sally, how are you feeling today?" The medical assistant asked Sally.

"I am doing good today. I had a few patients today to work on, but other than that, I am good." Sally responded.

The medical assistant took Sally to the back room to wait for the doctor. After about 20 minutes, the doctor came into the room.

"Hey Sally, how are you doing today?" Doctor asked.

"I am doing great, and I feel great, too," Sally responded.

"Well, that is good to hear. Now, let's get your physical done so you can return to your patients. I am sure they need you." The doctor said.

"That sounds good to me." She said.

As the doctor completed the physical, he told Sally he wanted to run a few routine blood tests. As he left the room, the medical assistant came in to do the blood work.

"Hi Sally, I will do your blood work for the doctor. Is that okay?" The medical assistant asked.

"Oh, are you new? I haven't seen you here before." Sally asked her.

"I just started a few days ago. The doctor hired me right out of school." She responded.

Sally looked nervous but decided to let her draw her blood. As the medical assistant put the needle in the arm, she realized she had missed the vein. No blood was going into the tube that was connected to the needle. At that moment, she began moving the needle around in the arm, hoping to find the vein. Sally started to feel a sharp, stinging sensation in her arm. Nevertheless, she didn't say anything to her. As the medical assistant continued to fish around in the arm, Sally's pain started to get worse and worse.

"It is starting to hurt now. I am feeling a sharp, stinging pain all over my arm. Please stop." Sally told her in a painful voice.

"Okay, I almost got it. Give me a second." She told Sally.

At that moment, blood began to flow into the tube, and she could get the blood the doctor ordered. She wrapped up Sally's arm and apologized for the discomfort. Sally said nothing, walked out of the office, and headed home for dinner. Her arm was in real pain.

When Sally got home, she put some ice on her arm, hoping to relieve the pain.

"Are you okay, honey?" Her husband asked.

"No, my arm is killing me from the blood draw." She responded.

"Maybe you are just sore. You will feel better in the morning." Her husband told her.

"I hope so. I have a lot of patients tomorrow." She said.

The following day, Sally could not fully move her arm. She had a hard time bending her arm without being in tremendous pain. At that point, she knew something was very wrong. She immediately left and went to see her doctor.

She told him about her arm when she arrived at her doctor's office. He examined her arm and realized she had nerve damage from the blood draw.

"I will need to run a few more tests, but it looks like there might be nerve damage to your arm." The doctor told her.

"Is it permanent? Will it heal in time?" She asked him.

"I am not sure. It could heal in time, or we might have surgery if it does not get better." He told her.

"What? Surgery? I have patients that need me. I cannot get surgery. There must be another way." She asked him.

"We just have to wait and see if it gets better. Then we can decide what to do." He told her.

Sally's life was turned upside down. She had to cancel her patients' appointments in the following weeks and hire a new dentist to take over for her. She had to have surgery and was on permanent disability. She could no longer practice dentistry. Her love for her work was gone. Her patients, who trusted only her to do their dental work, were forced to find another dentist. Their lives were also turned upside down because of a simple routine blood draw gone wrong.

WHAT HAPPENED?

It should be obvious as to what happened to Sally. When the medical assistant attempted to draw her blood and missed the vein, she began to fish and probe around Sally's arm, hoping to catch the vein. While moving the needle around in the arm, she hit a nerve.

Every needle used for a blood draw is like a tiny scalpel entering the arm. The needle tip is very sharp and can cut the tiny tissue fibers, a nerve, or an artery while probing or fishing around in the arm. The Clinical Laboratory Standard Institute, or CLSI, does not recommend manipulating the needle, or what is commonly called "fishing," while the needle is in the arm. Most undocumented needle injuries are due to "fishing" around the arm when a phlebotomist misses a vein. Internal bleeding can occur when an artery is punctured or lacerated from probing and fishing with a needle.

In the case of Sally, the nerve damage was irreversible, and Sally could no longer practice dentistry. The phlebotomist took away her family, that depended on her to provide for them. Sally's patients also suffered because Sally was the only dentist they trusted. Anybody who draws blood should never probe or fish in a patient's arm. CLSI recommends one option if the phlebotomist misses the vein. The person can move the needle further in the arm or pull it back a little. That is it.

Case #5: When Blood Kills

Jeff was a simple family man who worked 60 hours weekly to support his family. He was married for 12 years and had three kids. He managed a large bookstore in his city. Jeff was injured on the job and needed surgery. A few days before his surgery, the pain from the injury was too much for him to bear. He immediately went to the hospital, and they admitted him instantly.

"Good morning, Jeff. How are you feeling today?" The doctor asked Jeff as he entered his room.

Jeff was sharing a room at the hospital with another patient.

"I feel much better with the painkillers you gave me," Jeff responded.

"Well, do not get used to it. Those are only temporary until we do the surgery." The doctor told him.

"We should be able to do the surgery in the morning. I am going to order the blood work that is needed for the surgery. We need to make sure we have your blood type ready in case we need it." The doctor explained.

"No worries, doc, thank you," Jeff responded.

Jeff's family was also there to make sure he was okay and to make sure he did not need anything before his surgery in the morning.

"Okay, honey, we have your toothbrush, pajamas, and the fuzzy slippers you love." His wife told him.

"Thank you, babe. Where are the kids?" Jeff asked.

"Oh, I took them to your mother's house to play. I will get them some food right now and then return so they can see you before surgery tomorrow."

"Oh great, I missed them so much these last few days by not being home with them." He responded.

As Jeff's wife was leaving, the phlebotomist stood outside the room, preparing her supplies to draw Jeff's blood. She was busy most of the day running around the hospital. There was a shortage that day. Two other phlebotomists called off sick. She also had a few unlabeled tubes in her cart from another blood draw she had just finished.

"Good morning! I will take your blood for tests that your doctor ordered." The phlebotomist said while entering the room.

The phlebotomist started looking at Jeff's arm to see what vein she wanted to use. At that moment, the nurse walked into the room.

"Hey, can you also draw the patient in the next bed? Thanks." The nurse said very quickly, going in and out.

The phlebotomist finished drawing Jeff's blood and quickly went to the next bed to draw their blood. The phlebotomist quickly got the blood and headed out of the room and back to the lab.

The following day, the doctor entered Jeff's room to prepare him for the surgery.

"Okay, Jeff, we will get you down to the surgery room and get you ready. Do you have any questions?" The doctor asked.

"Nope. I am ready to go. Let us do this doc." Jeff responded.

During the surgery, Jeff's family was waiting in the waiting room. Jeff's wife was getting nervous as a few hours passed. Suddenly, the waiting room door opened, and the doctor came out quietly. He had a blank look on his face with no expression.

"Oh, hi, doctor. Is everything okay?" She asked.

The doctor took a moment before speaking.

"I am not sure what happened. Jeff reacted to the blood we gave him during surgery. I am sorry, Linda, but Jeff did not make it through surgery." The doctor responded.

Jeff's kids came running over to their mom in tears at that moment. Linda hugged them while they all cried, wondering what happened to their dad and husband.

WHAT HAPPENED?

Let us examine what happened when the phlebotomist came into Jeff's room to draw his blood. The phlebotomist had a busy day and was drawing blood from room to room. Two other phlebotomists called off sick that day, so she had to pick up extra draws.

While she was with Jeff, the nurse told her to draw the patient's blood next to Jeff's bed. The nurse gave no labels, so this was a verbal order for blood work. Both patients were scheduled for surgery.

The phlebotomist did both blood draws and went to the lab to get the missing labels. While she was there, she took all her labels and put them on the tubes, not realizing that she just mislabeled Jeff's tubes with the patient next to him.

Jeff received blood that was not his own. He received blood that belonged to the patient next to him. The phlebotomist failed to label all her tubes in front of the patient. The CLSI standard and practice is that every phlebotomist should label their tubes in front of their patients and have the patients verify the tube labels before the phlebotomist leaves their room. If the labels are unavailable, the phlebotomist needs to write the patient's information on the tubes in front of the patient and have them verify the information before leaving the room.

Jeff died because the phlebotomist failed to properly follow the basic standard and practice of labeling and verifying the tubes in front of a patient. Had the phlebotomist labeled all her tubes properly in front of her patients with verification, Jeff would be alive today and with his family.

Things To Remember

Phlebotomy can be a difficult job at times. They deal with so many different kinds of patients. Some are nice, while others are rude and mean. They deal with infants and geriatric patients who have hard veins to draw. Nevertheless, the most frustrating of all is that they are underpaid. Since 75 percent of all diagnostic results come from blood draws telling the doctor what is wrong with the patient, why would the phlebotomist who takes the blood sample be so underpaid?

There are so many things that can go wrong when drawing the blood. Without the phlebotomist, the lab cannot function properly. Furthermore, the hospital would have to shut down and lock its doors without the lab. The phlebotomist is among the most unappreciated and underpaid people in the hospital and lab today.

The phlebotomist needs to be adequately trained and valued by any facility. Every state needs to follow California's example and develop new regulations and laws that force phlebotomy schools to properly take the time to train every student under the governing agencies of phlebotomy. Those agencies are HIPAA, CLIA, CLSI, and OSHA. The standard of training should be the same as a nurse or even an LVN.

RESOURCES USED

Book Used

Phlebotomy Essentials, Ruth McCall, Jones & Bartlett Learning; 7th edition (July 4, 2020

Online Article Resource

Drawing Without a License

Phlebotomists Get Little Training, Regulation

By Ranit Mishori; Special to The Washington Post; Tuesday, June 1, 2004; Page HE01

Online Resources

American Society of Clinical Pathology https://www.ascp.org

Clinical Laboratory Improvement Amendments
https://www.cdc.gov/clia

Clinical Laboratory Standards and Institute
http://clsi.org

Health Insurance Portability and Accountability Act,
https://www.hhs.gov

A GUIDE

THAT WILL MAKE YOU A
SUCCESSFUL PHLEBOTOMIST

Often people wonder what the tips and tricks for a successful phlebotomist are. Do you know? 8 out of 10 successful people, on average, start from the mindset they have. The successful mindset of a phlebotomist is the initial guide to a successful career. Not only successful but also an educated person. What are the lessons that successful phlebotomists in this world have that make their lives more successful? Everything is wholly and thoroughly discussed in this book.

ABOUT THE AUTHOR

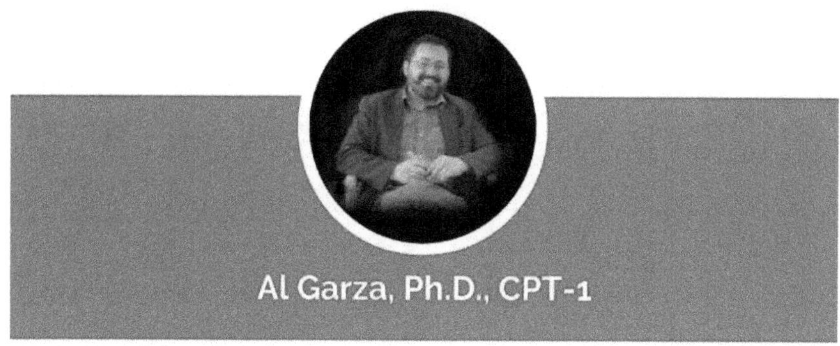

Al Garza has been a phlebotomist and an educator for 20 years. He currently owns Victor Valley Phlebotomy Training and Phlebotomy Solutions. He has taught thousands of students and helped dozens of individuals start their own phlebotomy school. He has also trained doctors and nurses on the fundamentals of phlebotomy. His experience and education make his book a valuable resource for any student or phlebotomist today.